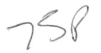
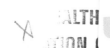

NURSE EDUCATION – THE WAY FORWARD

**PLEASE BE ADVISED THAT THIS BOOK IS
AN OLD EDITION, NO LONGER REQUIRED BY
THE LIBRARY.**

**THEREFORE THE INFORMATION MAY BE
OUT OF DATE.**

NURSE EDUCATION – THE WAY FORWARD

PHILIP BURNARD
MSc RGN RMN DipN CertEd RNT

Lecturer in Nursing Studies
School of Nursing Studies
University of Wales College of Nursing
Cardiff

CHRISTINE M CHAPMAN
OBE BSc(Hons) MPhil SRN SCM RNT FRCN

Formerly Professor of Nursing Education, and
Dean of the School of Nursing Studies
University of Wales College of Medicine
Cardiff

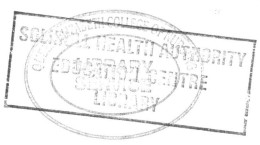
SCUTARI PRESS
London

© Scutari Press 1990

A division of Scutari Projects, the publishing company of the Royal College of Nursing

First published 1990

British Library Cataloguing in Publication Data
Burnard, Philip
  Nurse Education: The Way Forward
  1. Great Britain. Nurses. Professional education
  I. Title   II. Chapman, Christine M. Christine Murielo *1927–*
610.73071141

  ISBN 1–871364–34–5

Phototypeset by Input Typesetting Ltd, London
Printed and bound in Great Britain by
Biddles Ltd, Guildford and King's Lynn

Contents

Preface

Nurse education is constantly changing. At the time of writing this book it is undergoing very considerable change: curriculum modification, discussion and implementation of Project 2000, development of further and higher education in nursing.

Nurse Education: the Way Forward offers historical information, theory, practical ideas and opinion about a variety of aspects of nurse education. It is aimed at all those who are involved in the process of nurse education: students of various sorts, tutors and lecturers, nurse managers and clinical practitioners, and we hope that it will help to spark thought on and discussion of the topics that form its contents. It offers a broad canvas, which may serve to illustrate the events and ideas that have led to the present changes in nurse education, rather than a comprehensive treatment of the subject for which several first-class books have been written for the nurse educator.

The book is divided into three parts. Part I offers a review of the history of nurse education and shows how various people, laws and institutions have affected nursing education. Part II considers a variety of topical curriculum issues and explores them critically. Part III looks to the future and discusses new proposals and developments in the field, including Project 2000 and changes in both basic and higher nurse education.

We have both been teachers of nurses for a number of years, in basic, further and higher education. While our individual backgrounds and experiences are different and while we each have a different approach to nursing education, we are both committed to the further development of nurse education as a means of enhancing both nursing care and the nursing profession. We hope that this variety and diversity has contributed to a readable and useful book.

Philip Burnard
Christine Chapman
Cardiff 1990

PART I

Background and Context

CHAPTER 1

The Decision-makers

INTRODUCTION: THE EARLY DAYS

It is generally acknowledged that modern nursing owes its existence to Florence Nightingale and the establishment of the Nightingale School based at St Thomas' Hospital in London. However, it
is important to pay tribute to the work of Pastor Theodore
Fliedner, who established education for nurses in the Deaconess
Institute at Kaiserworth. There is no doubt that Florence Nightingale was greatly influenced by what she observed and learnt there,
as was Elizabeth Fry who, prior to the commencement of the
Nightingale School, started a small society of nurses to work
among the poor. While there does not appear to have been any
formal training given to this group of nurses, the influence of
Elizabeth Fry as a role model should not be underestimated. Other
religious groups gradually developed nurses, mainly to work in
the community, and eventually, in 1848, the Church of England
set out to reform hospital nursing by establishing St John's House,
from which probationers were sent to train at the Westminster
and Middlesex Hospitals and later at King's College Hospital, all
in London. These probationers had to pay a fee of £15 per annum
for their training, which lasted 2 years; at end of this time they
were officially recognised as nurses but had to work a further 5
years before they received a certificate (Abel-Smith, 1960).

Despite these and other developments, the first systematic attempt
to train nurses outside religious institutions was initiated by Florence Nightingale in 1860 with the establishment of the Nightingale
School. Her vision was that of a dedicated individual meeting the
physical and spiritual needs of the patient and assisting the doctor
in the curative task. Originally the probationers were recruited

3

from those with a minimum of educational requirements and the maximum of moral stature, although they had to be able to read medical books and write notes! Such pupils were expected to assist the doctor in the process of cure, acting as a skilled auxiliary constantly attending the patient as directed.

However, from 1867 the Nightingale School had two portals of entry: as ordinary probationers mentioned above, who got free training and maintenance, and as 'lady-pupils' who paid for their maintenance during training. It was clearly laid down that applicants for the 'lady' class of probationer had to 'desire to qualify themselves for superior situations', and there is little doubt that they fulfilled this criterion in that, by 1887, 20 hospitals, organisations and institutions had matrons or superintendents who had trained at the Nightingale School. Viewed historically, the Nightingale School was more important as a training school for matrons than as a training school for nurses. Ladies were sent there, 'with the special object that they should be passed on to be first, assistant superintendents and ultimately, heads of nursing departments in hospitals'. Interestingly, there was no great emphasis made on 'experience' and many of these ladies entered high office within a very short time of leaving the School.

Miss Nightingale had a very clear view of the role of these new matrons. Writing to one of them in 1867 she said, 'The whole reform in nursing both at home and abroad has consisted in this: to take all power out of the hands of the men, and put it in the hands of one female trained head and make her responsible for everything (regarding internal management and discipline) being carried out . . . Do not let the doctor make himself Head Nurse' (Abel-Smith, 1960). Needless to say, such a statement resulted in opposition from the medical staff, who feared that these educated women would undermine their authority, even though the nurses protested that as far as medical treatment was concerned they were there to carry out the doctors' orders. However, then, as now, it was difficult to draw the line between general nursing care, which came under the supervision of the matron, and medical treatment, which remained the sole responsibility of the doctor.

Unfortunately for the nursing profession there were always more 'ordinary' than 'lady' probationers and, therefore, the concept of the nurse as the doctor's assistant became the accepted role pattern. One of the effects of this perception was to link the activity of nursing to a medical model, the patient being seen as a repository of disease rather than as an individual, and this perception affected the pattern of nursing education and curriculum content until very recently.

THE DEVELOPMENT AND ROLE OF THE STATUTORY BODIES

The General Nursing Councils (GNCs)

The battle to achieve registration for nurses was long and hard, with the opposing sides being headed by two formidable ladies. For registration was Mrs Bedford Fenwick and against was Florence Nightingale. Those for registration, led by the British Nurses' Association, had as their aim 'to unite all British nurses in membership of a recognised profession and to provide for their registration in terms satisfactory to physicians and surgeons, as evidence of their having received a systematic training'. While this demonstrated a desire for nurses to be recognised as professionals in their own right, it still acknowledged the fact that nurses' practice was largely controlled by the medical profession. Meanwhile, the Hospitals' Association supported the views expressed by Florence Nightingale that 'devotion, gentleness, sympathy, qualities of overwhelming importance in a nurse, could not be ascertained by public examination'. This view still has its adherents today and often finds expression in an anti-intellectual approach to nursing education.

However, despite the battle, in 1919 three Nurses Registration Acts (one for each Ministry of Health in England and Wales, Scotland and Ireland) were passed by Parliament and Mrs Bedford Fenwick became the first name on the new Register in England and Wales – SRN 1.

The Acts were similar to each other and future discussion will focus only on that for England and Wales. It was a short document with the following aims:

1. The setting up of a corporate body called the General Nursing Council for England and Wales.
2. The establishment and maintenance by Council of a Register of Nurses, with five parts as follows:

   a. A general part.

b. A supplementary part for male nurses.
c. A supplementary part for nurses trained in the nursing of the mentally ill.
d. A supplementary part for nurses trained in the nursing of sick children.
e. Any other prescribed part.

3. To make rules in respect of its work concerning the Register, examinations, discipline, its meetings, committees and badge. It was also required to draw up rules governing the admission to the Register of existing nurses.
4. To allow for registration of certain nurses trained outside the United Kingdom.
5. To formulate an appeals procedure for any person aggrieved following removal of his or her name from the Register and for any institution refused approval as a nurse training school.
6. To state penalties that could be imposed by criminal courts on persons misusing the title 'Registered Nurse'.
7. To deal with personnel matters such as staffing and expenses.

The Act also specified the membership of the new Council as follows:

- Two people unconnected with medicine or nursing to be appointed by the Privy Council.
- Two people to be appointed by the Board of Education.
- Five people to be appointed by the Minister of Health.
- 16 to be nurses, appointed by the Minister of Health after appropriate consultation.

This constitution ensured a majority of nurses and was in accord with the desired aim of making nurses responsible for their own educational provision and standards.

The term of the new Council was to be 2 to 3 years, at the end of which the 16 new members were to be elected by the nurses on the Register.

The only point on which Mrs Bedford Fenwick did not achieve her declared aim was that the first chairman was not a nurse but a Mr J. C. Priestly, KC.

So began an era of decision-making, with many of the early

decisions still affecting nursing education today. For example, at their first meeting the Council decided that the minimum age of entry to the Register should be 18 years of age; that prior to registration the applicant would have to produce evidence of good character; and that there should be a division in the Mental Nurses Register to allow for the registration of 'nurses of mental defectives. The care of the mentally defective having been defined under the 1913 Mental Deficiency Act.'

Some decisions such as the setting up a Register for fever nurses have since been discontinued and others such as the formation of various committees were mainly related to the way in which the Council processed its work.

The Mental Nurses Register also had a difficult time as mental nurses had had their own national examination from 1891 and resisted any attempt at a 'take-over' by the GNC. It was not until after the Second World War that mental nursing really became integrated into the GNC structure.

The next Council with its 16 elected members continued to create the structure for the control of nursing education; for example they set up the Boards of Examiners and held the first examinations and commenced the inspection and approval of training institutions, and in 1924 the first nurse was removed from the Register following a conviction for felony. In 1926 Ellen Musson became the first nurse chairman of the GNC, and she was to retain that position for 18 years. It might fairly be said that nurses, via their representatives on the Council, were now in control of their own destiny.

The years passed and with them other changes occurred. For example, the Nurses Act 1943 allowed 'enrolment of assistant nurses for the sick'.

Following the Second World War there were a number of reports dealing with nursing matters such as wastage of nurses, the need to give learners student status, the provision of adequately trained teaching staff, and so on. Unfortunately, the fate of the recommendations of most of these reports, which have remarkable similarity, was rejection by the GNC as being unworkable. Perhaps this is not surprising when the nurse membership over the years is considered as, although elected, the nurses were not representative of the whole profession, being heavily weighted towards

London Teaching Hospital matrons. Their concern was quite naturally the staffing of their hospitals and this resulted in the educational needs of the learner being relegated to second place, despite being one of the main functions of the Council (White, 1985).

Further Nurses Acts followed; in 1949 the Council was reconstituted to have 17 elected members and 17 appointed members, six of the latter to be nurses. This meant that 23 of the 34 seats had to be held by nurses. The Act also set up Area Nurse Training Committees to advise and assist the Council and to administer the budget for nurse training, which, for the first time, was to be provided separately from the main hospital budget. The male part of the Register was merged into the main part, the annual retention fee for the Register was abolished and, following the initiation of the National Health Service (NHS), the Minister of Health became able to reimburse the cost of inspection and approval of training institutions. This enabled some of the deficiencies of training institutions to be tackled and, in addition, attention was focused on ways of attracting and training more nurse teachers.

The 1957 Act was one mainly consolidating the previous Acts, and in 1967 was amended by the Teachers of Nurses Act, which allowed the Council to admit as nurse tutors qualified teachers who were also nurses.

There were other minor Acts in 1961 and 1964 and the last Act relating directly to the GNC was that of 1969.

The role of a Statutory Body in maintaining standards by controlling education and training is an onerous one. From the start the GNC adhered to a medical model of nursing and hence education. This was clearly demonstrated by the emphasis on medical nursing, surgical nursing or other medical speciality divisions in both theoretical teaching and practical 'experience'. Although by 1969 the GNC's *Syllabus of Subjects for Examination and Record of Practical Instruction and Experience for the Certificate of General Nursing* (General Nursing Council, 1969) had headings such as 'Principles and Practice of Nursing', 'Study of the Human Individual', 'Concepts of the Nature and Cause of Disease' and 'Principles of Prevention and Treatment', which might suggest a broader outlook, Section 2 is devoted to 'Surgical Nursing', 'Gynaecological Nursing' and so on through a wide range of clinical specialities and Section 3 asks that the number of weeks spent in these areas of experience be specified. So this rigidity of approach over the years stifled development and perpetuated a medical orientation to nursing. This had the effect of emphasising nursing's subservient position to medicine, hindering movement toward self-determination, autonomy and professionalisation, despite the fact that outside the acute field nursing was and is frequently carried out with little contact with the doctor, and even in the acute areas medically prescribed care is only a small proportion of that provided by nurses over 24 hours.

This perception of the role of the nurse as being someone who merely obeys doctors' orders had the effect of reducing the amount of knowledge required by the nurse. What need is there of understanding if all that is required is the ability to follow instructions? It is not surprising that a strong anti-intellectual lobby developed in nursing and, indeed, to a lesser extent still exists today. Instead, emphasis is placed on 'experience', on the 'how' of nursing tasks rather than on the 'why' of nursing knowledge. Such an approach also supports the idea of learning by providing service. While an apprenticeship model of learning, which requires that each learner works with, and is taught and supervised by, an expert practitioner, can be an effective way of learning a practical skill, this situation has never obtained in nursing. On the contrary, the skilled practitioner has normally had a large number of learners to supervise, teaching has tended to be seen as the province of the 'school' and the learner's position as an employee and provider of service has been paramount. Such a situation emphasises task performance and results in things being done because of tradition rather than because of research-based knowledge showing that such action is beneficial for the patient.

The double role of 'learner' and 'service provider' has long been commented on as a source of conflict: 'That is where the difficulty arises, is it not, that the probationer is both a student and a worker in the hospital and the claims to some extent conflict' (House of Commons Select Committee on the General Nursing Council, 1905), and almost 70 years later:

> 'some of the problems arising in nursing education seem to us to be fundamental; the ambivalent positions of the nurse in training as both learner and worker.' (Report of the Committee on Nursing, 1972)

Of course, it can be argued, and frequently has been, that by constantly interacting with different individuals the nurse will learn how to interact with them and will 'pick up' nursing skills and a degree of knowledge on the way. Apart from the tautology of this argument, its inefficiency must be obvious. Trial and error learning is painful for both patient and nurse, is inefficient in time and unreliable in outcome, yet it is the pattern of nursing education that was perpetuated by the GNC from its inception, despite the pressure from many nurse educators and the findings of many reports on nursing.

Although 1969 saw the introduction of a new syllabus and also the first moves towards ward-based assessment, the break came in 1972 with the publication of the Report of the Committee on Nursing (Briggs Report), which re-emphasised many of the findings of previous reports and also a new devolved form of statutory control.

REFERENCES

Abel-Smith B (1960) *A History of the Nursing Profession*. London: Heinemann.
General Nursing Council (1969) *Syllabus of Subjects for Examination and Record of Practical Instruction and Experience for the Certificate of General Nursing*. London: GNC.

Acts of Parliament

Nurses Registration Acts 1919 (England and Wales; Scotland; Ireland)
Nurses Act 1943
Nurses Act 1949
Nurses Act 1957
Nurses Act 1961
Nurses Act 1964
Nurses Act 1969

Reports

Report of the Committee on Nursing (Briggs Report), 1972, Cmnd 5115. London: HMSO.
Report of the House of Commons Select Committee on the General Nursing Council, 1905.

FURTHER READING

White R (1976) Some political influences surrounding the Nurses Registration Act, 1919, in the UK. *Journal of Advanced Nursing,* **1**: 206–217.
White R (1978) *Social Change and the Development of the Nursing Profession. A Study of the Poor Law Nursing Service.* London: Kimpton.
White R (1985) *Political Issues in Nursing.* Chichester: John Wiley and Sons.

CHAPTER 2

The Development of Post-Registration (Post-basic) Education

HEALTH VISITING

The rapid move towards industrialisation in the nineteenth century highlighted the poverty and squalor of the living conditions of most of the country's working class. These conditions were reflected in the high infant mortality rate and were also seen in the poor physical condition of recruits to the army. It would appear from records that the first development towards what eventually became called health visiting occurred in 1852 with the setting up of the Manchester and Salford Reform Society. Visitors from the Society gave out tracts and hygiene information to the poor and eventually developed a form of health education. This increased with the appointment of sanitary visitors, who later became known as health visitors. It is interesting to note that these first visitors were not all nurses but included doctors, teachers and sanitary inspectors, yet the role was eventually seen to be most appropriately filled by a registered nurse and some councils also demanded that the nurse possess a midwifery qualification. The first training course was set up by no less than Florence Nightingale in the 1890s. She saw clearly the role for these visitors, stating:

> 'It hardly seems necessary to contrast sick nursing with this [health visiting]. The needs of home health require different, but not lower, qualifications and are more varied. She must create a new work and a new profession for women.'

By 1907 there were several forms of training available, ranging from a 2-year course for those with no nursing training to a 6-month course for the registered nurse. By 1919, with the establishment of the Ministry of Health, a common pattern emerged and

13

local councils were required to meet standards set jointly by the Ministry of Health and the Board of Education. In 1928 the Ministry of Health decreed that all health visitors must hold the certificate of the Royal Sanitary Association. Training was 6 months for registered nurses or midwives and 2 years for all others.

Emphasis was placed on the welfare of mothers and of children under 5 years of age, although there was some concern for the health of the school child.

Following the Second World War and the emergence of the welfare state, with its Acts covering all aspects of welfare of the population, the role of the health visitor expanded towards concern for the whole family. This had the result of producing some conflict with the role of the social worker as neither role was clearly delineated. In 1953 a working party was set up to survey the role of the health visitor and to examine ways in which recruitment could be improved. The report, named after its chairman as the Jamieson Report, made recommendations that led to the setting up of a Statutory Body to control the preparation of health visitors, and defined the role of the health visitor as one of 'health education and social advice' with regard to all members of the family and to the part played by other workers'.

As a result of the above report the Health Visiting and Social Work (Training) Act was passed in 1962. This Act set up joint councils for health visiting and social work training, with a single chairman. Subsequently, in 1970 these councils were separated and the Council for the Education and Training of Health Visitors emerged, its prime function being:

> 'to promote the training of health visitors by seeking to secure suitable facilities for the training of persons intending to become health visitors.'

The new syllabus that was produced by this body clearly built on the skills and knowledge acquired during basic general nurse training, despite a debate that continued regarding the suitability of preparation in the care of the sick as a basis for health education, health promotion and disease prevention.

DISTRICT NURSING

Like health visiting, district nursing in its present form is built on a basic nursing qualification. This has not always been the case, as the first systematic training to enable nurses to work in the community was probably that initiated by William Rathbone in Liverpool in 1862. In 1874 the National Association for Providing Trained Nurses for the Sick Poor in London and Elsewhere was founded and a year later published a report indicating the need for skilled nurses and the dangers inherent in amateur care. There was also an emphasis placed on the necessity of attracting well-educated women to care for the sick in their own homes, as it was felt that this type of care required greater personal responsibility and initiative than that required in hospitals where the discipline was greater and more easily enforced. In 1888 an institute (the Queen's Institute) was set up 'to promote the education of nurses for the sick poor in their own homes'. From such beginnings developed a number of other philanthropic organisations concerned with the care of the poor and the sick and these all produced training programmes. Many of these bodies had strong religious affiliations while others, particularly in the large cities, were under the control of the local authority.

Despite the early recognition of the need for special preparation for nurses caring for patients in their own homes, there has in more recent years been a constant debate as to the amount and type of preparation that such nurses require. In 1953 a working party set up to look at the training of district nurses said that only a little training was required for state registered nurses to work 'on the district' and that nothing extra was required for the state enrolled nurse! The reason given was that district nurses no longer worked in isolation but were subject to overall supervision by the local authority.

The Public Health Act 1969 enlarged the field of practice of district nurses by allowing them to work in places other than patients' homes. This enabled them to work in doctors' surgeries and to undertake more technical tasks, which required a change in their curriculum to ensure adequate preparation. This change in site of practice laid the foundation of the development of yet another category, that of practice nurse. Other changes in practice occurred as early discharge from hospital increased, as did the number of elderly in the community, and these factors helped to strengthen the argument that nurses in the community require specialist training.

The Panel of Assessors for District Nurse Training was set up in 1959 and re-constituted in 1979. Its terms of reference (applying to the whole of the British Isles and not just England and Wales) were:

> 'To advise Health Ministers on the standard of education and training for district nurses and on the provision of courses and to ensure on behalf of Ministers that such courses meet the standard approved by Ministers.'

The Panel consisted of 20 members representing district nursing teaching and management, medicine and general education, all of whom were appointed by Ministers of Health after consultation with appropriate bodies. Initially the Panel was housed in the Department of Health and Social Security but later moved to separate premises in an attempt to secure greater autonomy in line with the other nurse training bodies.

OCCUPATIONAL HEALTH NURSING

The first known trained nurse to work in industry was employed in 1878 by J & J Coleman, the mustard manufacturers of Norwich. Inspectors of factories were appointed under the Factory Act 1833 and in about 1893 they were required to take account of the health of women at work. Most of the women inspectors were trained as district nurses, although later some obtained the diploma of the National Health Society.

The first course for 'industrial nursing' was held jointly between the College of Nursing and Bedford College (University of London) in 1934 and an Industrial Nursing Certificate was awarded. Development was slow until the war, when in 1939 the Ministry of Labour and National Service asked the Royal College of Nursing to help to increase the output of industrial nurses. This resulted in a proliferation of courses, varying in length from 6 weeks to 3 months (those undertaking a 6-week course were not eligible to enter the examination). Following the end of the war a committee was set up under Judge Dale to advise on the integration of the Industrial Health Service with the National Health Service. The Report, published in 1950, stressed the importance of the work of the industrial nurse. In the same year the first joint International Labour Organisation/World Health Organisation Expert Committee on Occupational Health met. British nurses seized this new title and from 1952 the Royal College of Nursing Industrial Nursing Certificate was re-titled the Occupational Health Nursing Certificate.

The Employment Medical Advisory Services Act 1972 and the Health and Safety at Work Act 1974 further stimulated the appreciation of the need for occupational health nurses.

MIDWIFERY

The emergence of midwifery as a profession in its own right commenced in the nineteenth century and found its first overt expression in the first Midwives Act 1902. Prior to this midwives largely had their skills passed down, often from mother to daughter, and although there were attempts to develop well educated midwives by the issuing of a certificate by the Obstetrical Society of London (1872) and by the setting up in 1881 of the Midwives Institute, later to become the Royal College of Midwives, it needed legislation finally to secure adequate training and regulation of midwifery practice. The original Act related to England and Wales; Scotland passed a similar Act in 1915 and Ireland in 1918.

The main function of the 1902 Act was the protection of the public and this is reflected in the membership of the first Central Midwives Board, which was established under the Act. It consisted of nine members: four medical practitioners and five others, one of whom had to be a woman! There was no provision for direct midwifery membership. Nevertheless, out of the five unspecified members on the first Board, three were midwives. It was not until 1920 that it became mandatory to have four midwife members nominated by the Royal College of Midwives and two by the Secretary of State. Although membership of the Board was later increased to 17, the midwife membership remained the same.

The functions of the Board were to provide training and examinations and maintain and publish a Roll of Certified Midwives. Despite repeated attempts to control attendance at births it was not until the Midwives Act of 1936 that unqualified attenders and 'monthly nurses' were finally prohibited from attending women in childbirth.

An extra responsibility of the Midwives Board is that it is required to make rules to 'restrict within due limits the practice of midwives'. These rules not only control the day-to-day practice of midwives but also help to delineate the boundaries between midwifery and obstetrics.

Today the majority of midwives enter training following nurse registration; this may be due to the lengthening, in 1938, of direct entry training to midwifery, to 2 years. There are vigorous moves being made at present to increase this number of direct entrants. Direct entry training now lasts 3 years. The length of training for registered nurses was increased in 1983 to 18 months to bring it into line with the requirements of the European Community.

An important aspect of educational control is that since 1949 all midwives are required to undertake a refresher course every 5 years in order to ensure that practice methods are kept up to date. In addition, each year the midwife is required to notify her intention to practise and this enables a check to be kept on both the number of practising midwives (as opposed to those who have qualified but no longer practise) and also their educational needs.

OTHER AWARD-GIVING BODIES

Before proceeding further with the changes that ensued from the recommendations of the Briggs Report, it is important to consider the way in which control of post-basic education developed.

In the 1920s the British Tuberculosis Association was set up to ensure high standards of nursing in the care of patients with tuberculosis and diseases of the chest. This organisation conducted examinations and awarded a certificate. With the reduction in the number of cases of tuberculosis the Association changed its name to The British Thoracic and Tuberculosis Association, eventually dropping all reference to tuberculosis and becoming the British Thoracic Association, approving courses in the care of chest diseases and awarding a certificate.

The Central Council for the Care of Cripples set up a Joint Examination Board in 1935, becoming responsible for the training of nurses in orthopaedic nursing and awarding both a certificate and a diploma. Once again the name changed over the years to reflect changing patterns of disease and also public perception of the people affected, becoming the British Orthopaedic Association. Both the above bodies provided pre- and post-registration courses.

Much later, in 1950, the Midland Institute of Otology produced a post-registration programme in otolaryngological nursing. Not to be outdone, in 1952 the Ophthalmic Nursing Board was founded and set up training courses for both registered and enrolled nurses, issuing after 6 months' training a diploma for first level nurses and a certificate for second level nurses.

It is interesting to consider why these bodies developed and why there was felt to be a need for these specialist courses. While it is true that some of the nurses working in these specialist fields felt the need for a more formal training programme and qualification, it was the doctors in these disciplines who were the prime movers. Not only did they feel the need for more skilled nursing care as they developed specialist knowledge and techniques but they also saw that the inducement of training and another qualification would assist in recruitment to these areas.

It was largely this need to recruit nurses to specific areas of care using the 'carrot' of training that produced an explosion in special courses offered by individual hospitals. These courses varied in length even for apparently the same training, had no common examinations or standards and, in many cases, exploited those who entered the course in that they were used principally to provide service and any teaching given was largely fortuitous.

In 1963 a sub-committee of the Standing Nursing Advisory Committee was set up to advise on post-basic education for nurses and produced its report in 1966: *The Post-Certificate Training and Education of Nurses* (Central Health Services Council, 1966). The report restricted its recommendations to general hospital-based nurses up to the grade of ward sister, although it listed courses in psychiatric and other hospitals. It confirmed the fact that many courses on offer were not educational and were used mainly to recruit staff, and advised the setting up of a national body to control standards, etc. The report acknowledged the strength of medical involvement in the development of the courses and recommended widespread consultation with the medical professional and educational organisations in order to set up a national controlling organisation. The outcome was the establishment in 1970 of The Joint Board of Clinical Nursing Studies, with the following terms of reference:

'To consider and advise on the needs of nurses and midwives for post-certificate clinical training in specialised departments of the hospital service in England and Wales and to co-ordinate and supervise the courses provided as a result of such advice.'

In 1974 this remit was widened to include community nurses. Similar bodies were set up in Scotland (1972), while Northern Ireland Council already had as one of its functions, 'to provide or approve further education appropriate for Registered or Enrolled Nurses or Midwives'.

The Joint Board set up specialist panels to consider the need for courses and from them developed the outline curriculum. The training institutions then developed the detailed syllabus and that and the institution itself, including its clinical facilities, was then inspected by the panel for approval to run the course. The Joint Board provided a variety of awards, certificates, statements of competence or statements of attendance.

As a result of the establishment of the Joint Board most of the other award-giving bodies gradually phased out their involvement with nurses' training and this was finally achieved following the 1979 Nurses, Midwives and Health Visitors Act.

REFERENCES

Acts of Parliament

Factory Act 1833
Factory Act 1893
Midwives Act 1902 (England and Wales)
Midwives Act 1936
National Health Service Act 1947
Midwives Act 1951 (Consolidating Acts)
Health Visiting and Social Work (Training) Act 1962
Public Health Act 1968
Employment Medical Advisory Services Act 1972
Health and Safety at Work Act 1974
Nurses, Midwives and Health Visitors Act 1979

Reports

Report of the Committee of Enquiry on Industrial Health Services (Dale Report), 1950, Cmnd 8170. London: HMSO.

Report of a Working Party in the Field Work, Training and Recruitment of Health Visitors (Jamieson Report), 1956. London: HMSO.

Central Health Services Council (1966) *Post Certificate Training and Education of Nurses*. London: HMSO.

Report of the Committee on Nursing (Briggs Report), 1972, Cmnd 5115. London: HMSO.

Report of the Working Party on Midwives (Stocks Report), 1949. London: HMSO.

Report of a Working Party on the Training of District Nurses, 1955. London: HMSO.

FURTHER READING

Allan P and Jolley M (1982) *Nursing, Midwifery and Health Visiting since 1900*. London: Faber and Faber.

Nightingale F (1882) Letter to Mr Fredrick Varney. In a Report submitted to Buckingham County Council, 1911, pp. 17–19.

Joint Board of Clinical Nursing Studies (1979) *Notes on the Outline Curricula*. London: JBCNS.

Rathbone W (1890) *Sketch of the History and Progress of District Nursing from its Commencement in the Year 1859 to the Present Date*. London: Macmillan.

Slaney B (ed.) (1980) *Occupational Health Nursing*. London: Croom Helm.

Stocks M (1960) *A Hundred Years of District Nursing*. London: George Allen and Unwin.

CHAPTER 3

Reports, Acts and Directives

REPORT OF THE COMMITTEE ON NURSING, 1972

The Committee on Nursing was set up under the chairmanship of Professor (now Lord) Asa Briggs in 1970, with the following terms of reference:

'To review the role of the nurse and the midwife in the hospital and the community and the education and training required for that role, so that best use is made of available manpower to meet present needs and the needs of an integrated health service.'

The Report made 75 recommendations, all important, but for the purpose of this discussion only those with direct implications for nursing education will be considered. They can be dealt with under the headings listed below.

The Statutory Framework

1. There should be a single central body responsible for professional standards, education and discipline in nursing and midwifery in Great Britain – the Central Nursing and Midwifery Council.
2. There should be three distinct Nursing and Midwifery Education Boards for England, Scotland and Wales, responsible to the Council.
3. Midwifery interests should be represented by a statutory Standing Midwifery Committee of the Council. The Committee would advise Council and the Boards on midwifery education and have direct control of midwifery practice.
4. Below the three Education Boards there should be Area Committees for Nursing and Midwifery Education.

5. Responsibility for nursing and midwifery education should remain with the DHSS, SHHD and WO (Department of Health and Social Security, Scottish Home and Health Department and the Welsh Office).

Education

6. Education should be regarded as a continuing process under unified control.

7. Colleges of Nursing and Midwifery should be established throughout the country, financed through the Area Committees for Nursing and Midwifery Education.

8. The feasibility of setting up a number of Colleges of Health Studies should be explored.

9. Each College of Nursing and Midwifery should have a governing body with powers similar to those of governing bodies in institutions for which local education authorities are responsible.

10. Each College should be under a Principal with the assistance of a Vice-Principal (where necessary) and of lecturing and tutorial staff.

11. There should be close liaison for recruitment purposes between the Colleges and schools and the youth employment service.

12. There should be an increase in the number and the range of pre-nursing courses, with nursing cadet schemes continuing as part of that range, under the title Preparation for Nursing Courses.

13. At the point of entry to the nursing and midwifery profession, applicants should be drawn from a wide range of intelligence from average to highest. Suitability should not be determined by 'O' levels alone.

14. The age of entry should be reduced in two stages to 17½ in 1973 and to 17 in 1975.

15. There should be an annual national publication listing educational institutions and courses, similar to the King Edward's Hospital Fund for London Schools of Nursing Directory.

16. There should be one basic course of eighteen months for all entrants, which would lead to the award of a statutory qualification, the Certificate in Nursing Practice.

17. Courses should be planned on a modular basis and should include experience in general and psychiatric nursing of the various age groups in both hospital and the community. A defined amount of night duty should be part of the student's curriculum for its educational value only. No un-Certificated nursing student should be left in charge of the ward at night and there must be

proper support at night and at weekends in the clinical learning situation by teachers and senior staff.

18. The eighteen-month course leading to certification should be common to both prospective nurses and prospective midwives.

19. A further eighteen-month course, also on a modular basis and open only to those holding the Certificate in Nursing Practice, should be provided. It should lead to a secondary statutory qualification, Registration. The new Register, unlike the present Register, should not have separate parts.

20. For the more able students courses leading to Registration could include or be followed by courses leading to the award of a Higher Certificate (non-statutory) in a particular branch of nursing or midwifery.

21. There should be two ways of becoming a midwife:

a. following Registration as a nurse: a twelve-month course leading to Registration as a midwife and the award of a Higher Certificate.

b. following the Certificate in Nursing Practice: an eighteen-month course leading to Registration as a midwife and the award of a higher Certificate.

22. Examinations for the statutory qualifications of Certification and Registration should be supervised by the three Education Boards, who should use panels of internal and external assessors. The Boards should make a close study of examination and assessment techniques.

23. The Educational Boards should consider the best forms of educational provision:

a. for graduates entering nursing; and

b. in conjunction with universities, for students wishing to combine nursing with a degree.

24. Special training provision should also be made for mature entrants: these should take account of their domestic commitments.

25. Nursing students recruited overseas should be screened in their own countries wherever possible, and before beginning training they should be given effective orientation courses.

26. Post-registration courses, including clinical refresher courses, should be organised by the Education Boards as part of the on-going educational process.

27. There should be more 'back-to-nursing' and 'back-to-mid-

wifery' courses for qualified returners and 'keep-in-touch' courses for non-practising qualified nurses and midwives who might subsequently return.

28. There should be a planned in-service training scheme for nursing aides. The scheme should be based on a nationally agreed syllabus.

29. Students should continue to receive training allowances, which should be channelled through Area Education Committees, rather than student grants.

30. Nursing and midwifery education should include an introduction to the work of related professions such as the work of the professions supplementary to medicine and social work.

31. Educational and financial provision must be made in order that the nursing and midwifery profession shall become more research-based.

32. There should be improved continuity and co-ordination of education in the classroom and service, with greater involvement of teachers in the service setting and the use of, for example, clinically expert ward sisters and their community equivalents in Colleges.

33. It should be possible for people on the teaching staff of Colleges to hold honorary appointments in the service setting and vice versa.

34. Teachers of nursing and midwifery must be adequately prepared. They should no longer be required to teach all subjects on the syllabus. The basis qualification for teachers should be a one-year course for the Diploma in Nursing and Midwifery Education.

35. There should be a major drive, started as quickly as possible, to produce more nursing and midwifery teachers.

36. In liaison with the Education Departments, the Health Departments and the Central Council through its Education Boards should plan urgently a ten-year programme to increase those holding the Diploma and to qualify more teaching staff generally.

37. There should be refresher courses for teaching staff, taking account of newly identified needs as they arise.

While these are the main recommendations with direct implication for nursing and midwifery education, many of the others, under such headings as manpower, conditions of service, etc., have less direct effect.

As so often seems to have happened with reports regarding nursing, other things intervened; the Government was preoccupied until 1974 with a reorganisation of the health service and, therefore, despite pressure from the nursing profession to take action, nothing happened until 1977 when the Briggs Co-ordinating Committee was set up. The purpose of this committee was to seek agreement on the main areas of the Report in order to prepare legislation to lay before Parliament. This consensus was difficult to achieve. The various groups within nursing felt that they required special consideration and/or protection and there was much lobbying of members of Parliament both prior to the Bill being formulated and during its passage through the committee stages and the House. The result of this was to delay legislation, and the Bill finally received Royal Assent in the last hour of Parliament prior to its being prorogued for a General Election.

NURSES, MIDWIVES AND HEALTH VISITORS ACT 1979

The main recommendations of the Act were as follows.

Statutory Structure

The United Kingdom Central Council for Nursing, Midwifery and Health Visiting (UKCC). The membership is 45 persons, made up as follows:

- Five to be nominated from each of the four National Boards (In 1983 this number was increased to seven.)

  a. Two practising nurses.
  b. One practising midwife.
  c. One practising health visitor.
  d. One person engaged in the teaching of nursing, midwifery or health visiting.

- Seventeen Secretary of State nominations. These to be made after consultation with the appropriate bodies and to include registered medical practitioners, representatives from general education and other fields and other nurses, midwives or health visitors as required to ensure that the Council is able to fulfil its functions by having available the appropriate expertise.

Membership is for 5 years. The first Chairman, a nurse, was a

Secretary of State appointment; subsequently the Chairman is elected by and from among the Council's membership.

In order to achieve transfer from the old Statutory Bodies there was an initial period of 'shadow bodies' working towards the hand-over.

The Council has a Chief Executive and other professional and supporting staff to enable it to carry out its functions. Functions of the Council are:

1. The principal functions of the Central Council shall be to establish and improve the standards of training and professional conduct for nurses, midwives and health visitors.
2. The Council shall ensure that the standards of training they establish are such as to meet any community obligation of the United Kingdom.
3. The Council shall by means of rules determine the conditions of a person's being admitted to training, and the kind and standard of further training to be undertaken, with a view to registration.
4. The Rules may also make provision with respect to the kind and standard of further training available to persons who are already registered.
5. The powers of Council shall include that of providing, in such a manner as it thinks fit, advice for nurses, midwives and health visitors on standards of professional conduct.
6. In the discharge of its functions the Council shall have proper regard for the interests of all groups within the professions, including those with minority representation.

The Council was required to set up a standing committee for midwifery and also one for finance. In addition, the Secretary of State set up, with the Boards, a joint committee for health visiting and, although not required in the primary legislation, one was set up for district nursing. These committees have an important role in that Council or, in the case of the joint committees Council and the Boards, are required to consult them about matters concerning midwifery, health visiting or district nursing.

The National Boards

Four National Boards – for England, Wales, Scotland and Northern Ireland respectively – were set up under the Act. Maximum membership for Northern Ireland was 35 and for the other Boards 45.

Initially this membership was entirely nominated by the Secretary of State, until the Council had time to establish an electoral scheme. This came into effect in 1983 and varied the membership in that the Boards for Northern Ireland and Wales have 34 members, of whom 24 are elected and 11 appointed; Scotland has 25 elected and 12 appointed members; and England, with a Board of 45, has 30 elected and 15 appointed members. Council is responsible for holding the election for membership of the Boards, which is designated as follows:

Wales, Scotland and Northern Ireland each have elected in categories, 16 nurses, 4 midwives, and 4 health visitors, while England has 20 nurses, 5 midwives and 5 health visitors. The electorate are all persons on the Council's register. The remaining membership of the Boards is nominated by the Secretary of State after consultation and includes medical practitioners, educationalists and nurses from minority groups who might otherwise not have representation.

Functions of the National Boards
The Act states that: The National Boards shall in England, Wales, Scotland and Northern Ireland respectively:

'a. provide, or arrange for others to provide, at institutions approved by the Board:

i. courses of training with a view to enabling persons to qualify for registration as nurses, midwives or health visitors or for the recording of additional qualifications in the register; and
ii. courses of further training for those already registered;

b. ensure that such courses meet the requirements of the Central Council as to their content and standard;
c. hold, or arrange for others to hold, such examinations as are necessary to enable persons to satisfy requirements for registration or to obtain additional qualifications;
d. collaborate with the Council in the promotion of improved training methods; and
e. carry out investigations of cases of alleged misconduct with a view to proceedings before the Central Council or a committee of the Council for a person to be removed from the register.'

To summarise the functions of the Statutory Bodies: the Council decides on the standard that must be achieved before a person is admitted to the Register and retains the power to remove a person from that Register; and the National Boards approve forms of education and training and also the institutions in which they take place so that persons may be appropriately prepared to enter the Council's Register, and investigate cases where removal from the Register may be in question.

In 1988 a firm of management consultants, Peat Marwick McLintock (Peat Marwick McLintock, 1989) was asked by the Department of Health to review the work of the Statutory Bodies. Their recommendations, which are now out for consultation, suggest that:

1. elections from the profession should be to the UKCC not the National Boards. This would enable the UKCC to be directly accountable to the profession. Two-thirds of the membership should be elected and one-third appointed;
2. the UKCC should combine both the investigatory and the disciplinary functions;
3. the National Boards should become smaller, appointed executive bodies with closer links with their sponsoring and financing bodies – the Government departments in the respective countries. Members should be appointed for their expertise rather than representational interests.
4. the Boards should manage and finance both pre- and post-registration nursing and midwifery education.

There are also recommendations that are specific to the individual National Boards.

These suggestions are radical and require new primary legislation. At the time of writing no decisions have been made.

THE EUROPEAN COMMUNITY (EC)

As part of the agreement within the EC to allow freedom of movement and employment between the member countries a number of directives have been issued relating to the standard of education and training required by a variety of professional groups.

The Standing Committee of Nurses of the EC

The above Committee had its first formal meeting in Brussels in 1971. Membership is representative of the member countries of the EEC and nomination is made via the nurses' professional association, which is in membership of the International Council of Nurses (in the UK this is the Royal College of Nursing). The first directive concerning nurses responsible for 'general care' came into operation in June 1979 and was followed in the UK by the Nursing Qualifications (EEC Recognition) Order 1979. The first directive was concerned with the mutual recognition of diplomas. The second directive specified five essentials to be tested by examination. These were:

1. adequate knowledge of the sciences on which nursing is based;
2. sufficient knowledge of the nature and ethics of the profession and of the general principles of health and nursing;
3. adequate clinical experience under the supervision of qualified staff;
4. ability to participate in the training of health personnel;
5. experience of working with other professions in the health sector.

An annex to the second directive set out a brief outline of the content of the training, which is to be 3 years or 4600 hours in three main theoretical areas: nursing, basic sciences and social sciences. Practical instruction was to cover experience in seven areas: medical and surgical nursing, child care and paediatrics, maternity care, mental health and psychiatry, care of the old and geriatrics, and home nursing.

A further directive established an Advisory Committee on Training in Nursing to help to ensure a high and comparable standard of nursing education throughout the EC. Membership is of three experts from each member country: one from the practising profession, one from establishments providing training for nurses and one from the competent authority (that is the registering body, e.g. the UKCC).

EC directives on Training in Midwifery

A Permanent Committee of Midwives of the EEC was set up in 1967 and similar directives, coming into operation in 1983, have been issued for midwives. The main provisions are:

1. For direct entrants to midwifery training, the course should be 3 years full time.

2. For registered general nurses who conform to the nursing directives of the EC the UK has two options;
   a. a full-time 2-year training or 3600 hours; or
   b. a full-time training of 18 months or 3000 hours, and an additional year of practice.

The Nursing and Midwifery Qualifications (EEC Recognition) Order 1983 revoked the 1979 Nursing Qualification (EEC Recognition) Order 1979, so that changes that occurred as a result of the 1979 Nurses, Midwives and Health Visitors Act could be accommodated.

NURSING IN HIGHER EDUCATION

As stated earlier, some types of nursing education, e.g. health visiting, have been located in institutions of higher education for a considerable number of years. Since the 1950s more and more courses have moved into this sector and nurses may now enter the profession via a degree in nursing or may obtain a diploma and/or degree following registration. While any course that leads to entry on the UKCC's Register will require approval from the appropriate National Board, the institution will also have its own validating body that assures comparability with other academic courses. In universities in the UK this will be via the individual university's Academic Board, and in polytechnics the validating body is the Council for National Academic Awards (CNAA). While these two forms of validation normally take place separately, using different criteria, there are moves to achieve a joint validation process, thereby cutting down on duplication of time and effort.

WHO ARE THE DECISION-MAKERS?

The answer to this question is not as simple as it might have seemed when first asked. History has demonstrated the importance of individuals in the setting up and initial development of nursing training in all its aspects. While most of these individuals were nurses, there is evidence to suggest that medical practitioners often played a large part in the decision process and, on other occasions, political expediency may have been the driving force. Certainly the medical profession has always had a major role in decisions made regarding nursing education and it is only since the 1979 Nurses, Midwives and Health Visitors Act that their representation on Statutory Bodies has been reduced to reasonable levels. (It may be interesting to consider the fact that nurses do not have any influence 'as of right' on bodies concerned with medical education; the fact that one nurse at present sits on the General Medical Council is fortuitous, she is there as a lay member.)

The Statutory Bodies obviously play the most significant part in decisions regarding nursing education as they have to approve courses for registration, although within broad guidelines there is a degree of flexibility available for the training institutions.

General education also exerts a degree of pressure, not only via those courses based in higher education but also because the education received by the entrants to courses will, or should have, a bearing on the content and method of teaching.

Finally, the Government exerts pressure by its manpower requirements and other political policy decisions and by the fact that much of the time it controls the finance. (An interesting and important step to modify this latter point was taken when the UKCC decided to become self-financing.) This is particularly relevant following the recent publication by the Government of the White Paper *Working for Patients*. The possible impact of self-governing hospitals on nursing education has yet to be fully explored despite the Government's assurance that nursing and midwifery education will be protected.

All this may make it appear that nurses have very little control over their own education. This need not be so. First, membership of Statutory Bodies is largely by election and this mechanism can be used to ensure that a specific voice is heard. Examples of this have been seen in elections where tactical voting has been employed to ensure representation of minority groups. Second, the Statutory Bodies are required to consult the profession on major issues (compare the consultation over the proposals of Project 2000). This mechanism enables modifications to be made to proposals before they become enshrined in legislation. Finally nurses are voters and as such are able to lobby MPs, as was done, very successfully, prior to the passing of the 1979 Act, and they could, if organised, have an impact at the time of Parliamentary elections. If nurses used their power on the occasions of Parliamentary elections, they could also become a powerful lobby.

There is, therefore, no one answer to the question 'Who are the decision-makers?', but the profession could ensure that the reply is 'Mainly nurses'.

REFERENCES

Peat Marwick McLintock (1989) *Review of the United Kingdom Central Council and the Four National Boards for Nursing, Midwifery and Health Visiting*. London: Peat Marwick McLintock.

Working for Patients, Government White Paper on the National Health Service, 1989.

Acts/Orders of Parliament

Nursing Qualifications (EEC Recognition) Order, January 1980.
Nursing and Midwifery Qualifications (EEC Recognition) Order, 1983.

Report

Report of the Committee on Nursing (Briggs Report, 1972, Cmnd 5115). London: HMSO.

FURTHER READING

Official Journal of the European Communities, July 1977.
Quinn S (1980) *Nursing in the EEC*. London: Croom Helm.

PART II

Curriculum Issues

CHAPTER 4

The Nature of Nurse Education

EDUCATION OR TRAINING?

The words 'education' and 'training' are sometimes used synonymously. For example, it is not unknown for the building in which nurses receive instruction to be known as either the Nurse Training School or the Nurse Education Centre. Often, the latter is thought preferable.

As with any attempt to define words the best we can do is to offer a *stipulative* definition. That is to say that we can suggest how *we* are using words. There are, after all, no absolute meanings for words for, as Wittgenstein pointed out, 'meaning is use'. To discover what a word means we must look to see how it is being used. Clearly, we are not helped when we look at the use of the words in the above two descriptions of schools of nursing.

In a general way, however, it seems likely that the word 'training' is usually associated with a well-defined course with a definite end point and with an emphasis on the development of certain pre-defined skills. It can be said to be a convergent process in that all those undertaking it will end up with mostly the same skills and abilities. Education, on the other hand, is a divergent process of developing knowledge, skills, interests, values and so on. The aim of education is not some predetermined point, nor even the accumulation of particular knowledge and skills, but more the development of a critical ability and the means of becoming more and more flexible and adaptable. In this respect education has no end product – we can never say that we are 'educated'. It follows, too, from this definition that we cannot anticipate what an educated person will be like, for those in the process of being educated will always be in a state of becoming, a state of flux.

These two stipulative definitions may help us in the consideration of aims of nurse education. It may be argued that nursing has worked with a training model up until very recently. The aim has been to produce a 'standard nurse' who has certain skills and abilities that have been identified for her prior to her commencing her course. To become that nurse, she must submit herself to a very particular course of training, organised and presented for her by her nurse tutors. In this model it is not too difficult to identify the 'ideal type' of nurse, to develop a curriculum to produce such a person and then to run the course.

With education, however, the situation is different. If the person becoming educated is always in a state of becoming and has never 'arrived', it will be much more difficult to set down parameters for a course in nursing. Further, if by definition educated people vary from one another in fairly fundamental ways, it will be even more difficult to decide on the content and methods of such a course. One answer to this problem may lie in the notion of *negotiation*, a concept that will be under discussion at various points in this book. Suffice to say at present that the concept of negotiation, as it is being used here, involves at least the following criteria:

1. The student will have some autonomy in deciding her own course.
2. The tutor will have some say in what does and does not go into such a course.
3. The student and tutor will meet to discuss the content, methods and evaluation procedures that will be in the course.
4. There will be agreement between student and tutor about the nature and content of the course.
5. The course will satisfy an outside body responsible for maintaining a list of registered nurses.

It is not suggested that these criteria constitute necessary and sufficient criteria for satisfying the concept of negotiation but they do serve to point to the fact that negotiation is a *two-way* process. In recent years it has been tempting to think, in some quarters, that nurse education should become wholly student centred and that the tutor has somehow become a rather unnecessary appendage! It is acknowledged here that in true negotiation it must be clear that that negotiation develops from both sides and that there will always be areas that *are* negotiable and areas that are *not*. To think that everything in a curriculum can or should be negotiable is anarchical and unlikely to lead to a satisfactory educational experience for either student or tutor. Indeed, in the next chapter we will explore the degree to which *content* of a course *can* be negotiated.

Having identified some of the differences between training and education, we may now turn to consider different sorts of education as a means of further clarifying how it may be possible to make educational decisions in nurse education.

TWO APPROACHES TO EDUCATION AND LEARNING

The approach to learning suggested in this book suggests a certain view of education. This view is best articulated by a series of comparisons between two types of curriculum model. The two types are illustrated in Figure 4.1, which offers two 'ideal types' of curriculum: the classical and the romantic. This distinction has been made by a variety of writers, including the novelist Robert Pirsig (1974) and the educationalist Dennis Lawton (1973), who uses them to make comparisons between types of curriculum in a similar manner to that described here.

Classical model	Romantic model
1. Aims and objectives predetermined by teaching staff	1. Aims and objectives negotiated with students
2. Teaching methods chosen by teaching staff	2. Learning methods chosen by students in collaboration with teaching staff
3. Evaluation by tests and examinations	3. Self- and peer evaluation
4. 'Teaching from above'	4. Shared responsibility for learning

Figure 4.1 Two models of education and of the curriculum

It is suggested that the two curriculum models offer two different views of the nature of education and a closer examination of the two may help to illustrate this. The classical model is teacher- or tutor-centred: the teacher is a more important figure than the learner in that he plans and executes the programme. The teacher is the 'one who knows' and the student is the 'one who comes to learn'. The romantic model, on the other hand, is student-centred and its main aim is learning. In this model the teacher acts as a resource or as a 'facilitator of learning' (Rogers, 1983). A facilitator is not a teacher but one who helps others to learn for themselves.

In the classical model aims and objectives are predetermined by the teacher. Lessons are preplanned independently of the students. In the romantic model aims and objectives are negotiated with the learners: students' needs and wants are identified and learning sessions are then developed around those needs and wants.

In the classical model teaching methods are also predetermined by the teacher. In the romantic model they are chosen through collaboration with the learners, and participation in the learning process is voluntary. There is usually also an accent on *activity*: the learner is encouraged to take an active part in her own learning process.

Evaluation of learning in the classical model is by tests and examinations set by the teacher or by an outside examining board. In the romantic model both facilitator and learners engage in self- and peer evaluation (Kilty, 1981; Burnard, 1987). These approaches to evaluation enable the learner to assess her own performance and to receive feedback from both the facilitator and the other people in her learning group. In this way, she receives a 'triangulated' form of evaluation: she has three sets of perceptions of her learning instead of one.

It may be noted that the classical model involves 'teaching from above' whereas the romantic model is more concerned with the 'education of equals' (Jarvis, 1983). In the romantic model students and facilitator are 'fellow travellers', for, as we saw in Figure 4.1, the view of knowledge offered in this model is relative. There are no absolute truths or facts but views of the world are negotiated through discussion, argument and debate. Because each person's view of the world is different, so individual people's 'knowledge' will be different. In the classical model knowledge is not relative:

there are objective facts out there in the world that are subject to apprehension by those who seek them – a view of knowledge that can be traced back at least to Plato. Within this model it is the teacher's task to pass on those objective facts. In the classical model knowledge is 'impartial' and is unchanged by the one who knows it (Peters, 1966). In the romantic model knowledge is dynamic, ever-changing and very much a part of the one who does the knowing.

A similar distinction between two approaches to education is made by Freire (1972), who described the 'banking' concept of education versus the 'problem-posing' concept. The banking concept (which Freire argues is the traditional and predominant one) involves the teacher helping to fill his students with knowledge, which is later 'cashed out', relatively unchanged, in examinations. In this model 'more knowledge' is usually synonymous with 'better educated'. Alternatively, Freire's problem-posing approach to education is a means of education through dialogue. Facilitator and students meet and exchange ideas and experiences through critical argument and debate. Neither facilitator nor student has the 'right' answer; there is room for 'multiple realities' – different views of the world built on different experiences of that world.

Blaney (1974) summarises the more traditional teaching and learning relationship by reference to a variety of typical criteria, including the following:

- *Authority* is assumed by the educational institution and is largely external to the learners.
- *Objectives* are determined prior to the educational encounter and these provide the basis for programme planning and evaluation. These objectives are consistent with the aims of the providing agency, although they may be revised by the teacher.
- *Methods of instruction* are chosen for their demonstrated effectiveness in achieving the previously determined objectives.
- *The teacher's roles* are those of instructional planner, manager of instruction, diagnostician, motivator and evaluator.
- *The learner* assumes a dependent role regarding learning objectives and evaluative criteria; the learner's task is to achieve the prescribed objectives.
- *Evaluation* is criterion referenced, and criteria are based on the achievement of the prescribed objectives. The purpose of evaluation is to assess the effectiveness of instruction in

assisting learners to achieve the prescribed objectives, to improve the programme, and to diagnose learning difficulties.

These, then, are two ideal types of curriculum. What may make nurse education different from certain other types of education (including university education) is that nurses are required to follow a certain syllabus, laid down in the first instance by the Nurses, Midwives and Health Visitors Rules Approval Order (1983) and then by the National Boards. In the next chapter we explore the issue of content and discuss the degree to which curriculum content in nursing is prescribed and the degree to which it can be negotiated.

Underpinning the distinctions made here between two types of curriculum (and developed further in the next section on adult learning) is the issue of power. In the traditional, classical curriculum power was both held and exercised by the tutor or lecturer. It was the educators who decided on what should be learned, how it should be taught and what criteria should be used to determine to what degree learning had taken place. It is arguable, too, that they also decided what was to be *considered* as knowledge. Many nurses trained under such a system came to believe that what they were taught by their tutors was the truth, that the tutor's view of the world represented an accurate view. That was until they arrived in the clinical setting where they found that the tutor's view no longer necessarily held up. Indeed, the school of nursing/clinical nursing dichotomy has been researched and written about widely. Even faced by an apparent contradiction of 'truths', learners within the traditional system had little leeway to question what they were taught in the school of nursing because, as we have noted above, that system did not allow such questioning to take place. All the time that knowledge was handed down from tutor to learner, the question of the relativity of knowledge did not crop up. It is possible to question, also, the degree to which tutors in that system were aware of their own lack of critical awareness. When a person is immersed in a particular situation it is often difficult for him to realise that he is in it. A particular type of 'false consciousness' prevails.

With the push towards nurse educators furthering their own education and with the increasing emphasis on nursing moving towards a degree-based profession, it is possible to anticipate a further move in the direction of the relative and negotiable curriculum described here. Then, hopefully, the learner nurse will no longer be encouraged to store away undigested chunks of knowledge (Sartre referred to this sort of educational process as the 'digestive' approach) that she believes will serve her well throughout her nursing career. Instead, she will come to view knowledge as always and only tentative in nature – always subject to revision in the light of new evidence. The change will not come quickly. There is a long tradition in nursing of the sanctity of nursing knowledge and of the purity of knowledge gained from related disciplines. One example of this is the frequency with which a concept such as Maslow's hierarchy of needs (Maslow, 1972) is taught and espoused, without question, as a basis for understanding the needs of human beings. Only rarely are questions asked about the basis for the hierarchy, whether or not needs really are hierarchical in nature or whether or not the hierarchy has been subject to research. Perhaps it is through the development of research in nursing that change will occur although, again, it seems likely that such change will come slowly. Only recently a colleague of one of the present writers was recommended by a director of nurse education to 'go away and get the research bug out of your system'. It seems likely that familiarity and acceptance of research as an approach to learning will take time to become the norm.

ADULT LEARNING

The American educator Malcolm Knowles has used the term 'andragogy' to describe negotiated adult learning, as opposed to 'pedagogy' or teacher-directed, child education (Knowles, 1980). Knowles argues that negotiated and experiential learning are those types of education best suited to adults because:

- '● adults both desire and enact a tendency toward self-directedness as they mature, although they may be dependent in certain situations;
- ● adults' experiences are a rich resource for learning. Adults learn more effectively through experiential techniques of education such as discussion or problem-solving;
- ● adults are aware of specific learning needs generated by real life tasks or problems. Adult education programmes, therefore, should be organised around 'life application' categories and sequenced according to learners' readiness to learn;
- ● adults are competency based learners in that they wish to apply newly acquired skills or knowledge to their immediate circum-

stances. Adults are, therefore, 'performance centred' in their orientation to learning.'

All of these aspects of adult learning are appropriate in the teaching and learning of nursing. All learners coming to nurse education do so as adults; whatever criteria are used to measure adulthood it would be difficult to argue otherwise. They all bring to the learning situation a wealth of personal and occupational experience: no learners in nursing arrive as *tabula rasa* or 'blank slates'. All nurses, too, need to use the skills they learn for practical purposes within their lives and within their jobs. So, too, they need to apply what they learn in practical settings. All of these aspects of adult learning are also consistent with the learning approaches described throughout this book in that they emphasise the use of a balance between knowledge, practice and personal experience as the keystone of learning nursing.

Knowles et al (1984) have identified seven components of andragogical practice that they feel are replicable in a variety of programmes and training workshops throughout the world. These components are highly relevant to the development of nursing skills and nursing knowledge:

'• Facilitators must establish a physical and psychological climate conducive to learning. This is achieved physically by circular seating arrangements and psychologically by creating a climate of mutual respect among all participants, by emphasising collaborative modes of learning, by establishing an atmosphere of mutual trust, by offering to be supportive and by emphasising that learning is pleasant.
• Facilitators must involve learners in mutual planning of methods and curriculum directions. People will make firm commitments to activities in which they feel they have played a participatory, contributory role.
• Facilitators must involve themselves in diagnosing their own learning needs.
• Facilitators must encourage learners to formulate their own learning objectives.
• Facilitators must encourage learners to identify resources and to devise strategies for using such resources to accomplish their objectives.
• Facilitators must help learners to carry out their learning plans.
• Facilitators must involve learners in evaluating their learning, principally through the use of qualitative evaluation modes.'

Out of this discussion on the philosophical underpinnings of two approaches to the curriculum arise certain practical considerations for programme planning for nurses' training and educational courses. Brookfield (1986) discusses what he calls the principles of practice in community action projects. These principles, listed below, may well serve as the underlying principles for developing curricula for the training and education of nurses:

- '• The medium of learning and action is the small group.
- • Essential to the success of efforts is the development of collaborative solidarity among group members. This does not mean that dissension is silenced or divergence stifled; rather, group members are able to accept conflict, secure in the knowledge that their peers regard their continued presence in the group as vital to its success.
- • The focus of the group's actions is determined after full discussion of participants' needs and full negotiation of all needs, including those of any formal 'educators' present.
- • As adults undertake the actions they have collaboratively agreed upon, they develop an awareness of their collective power. This awareness is also felt when these adults renegotiate aspects of their personal, occupational and recreational lives.
- • A successful initiative is one in which action and analysis alternate. Concentrating solely on action allows no time for the group to check its progress or alter previously agreed-upon objectives. But if the members of the group engage solely in analysis, they will never come to recognise their individuality and collective power. Empowerment is impossible without alternating action and reflection.'

If Knowles and Brookfield are right, adults need to use what they learn. All learning about nursing needs to be grounded in the participants' practical experience and any new learning needs to be the sort that can be applied on future occasions. Both Knowles' and Brookfield's notions of the educational principles of facilitating learning groups are entirely relevant to the running of learning groups for nurses in that all learners coming to such groups (regardless of their status and of the specific discipline) are adults.

It is interesting to debate the degree to which all of the principles discussed so far can be brought into play in the development of a nursing curriculum. On the one hand, all nurse learners are adults, on the other, there is a statutory responsibility laid upon schools of nursing to ensure that all learners develop certain competencies – a restraint that is missing from many other adult educational courses.

The term 'curriculum' has been used to describe all the planned and unplanned activities that go to make up the educational process. Thus a curriculum is concerned with aims and objectives, teaching and learning methods, content to be taught and learned and evaluation methods. While the principles underlying curriculum development in nursing have been described extensively elsewhere (Henderson, 1982; Allan and Jolley, 1987; Davis, 1987; Greaves, 1987), it is notable that the principles of andragogy, as described here, can be used in the process of curriculum development in that they suggest that the nurse as an adult learner should play an active part in each stage of the curriculum process. The *degree* to which she can do that is discussed in Chapter 5.

WHERE DO NURSES LEARN NURSING?

Nurses, of course, learn in both the formal, classroom setting and in the clinical and community arena. It is important that all learners appreciate the need to consider both settings. Chapter 7 on experiential learning can be applied as much to clinical learning as to classroom learning. It is notable that in a recent study of nursing students' views of experiential learning (Burnard, 1989) all the learners interviewed made a distinction between experiential learning as a series of exercises carried out in the school of nursing and experiential learning as 'learning through doing' in the clinical setting. It is notable, too, that those students talked of learning in the clinical setting as being more 'real' than that which occurred in the classroom.

A number of studies have identified the apparent split between theory and practice in nurse education (Powell, 1982; Melia, 1983), and it is not intended that the arguments surrounding this split be rehearsed here. Suffice to say that those involved with nurse education should be prepared to make full use of clinical learning. One way of doing this is via the negotiated curriculum. If learners are encouraged to discuss their clinical experience once they return to the school of nursing, and that experience is then used to determine the learning programme for that week, a synthesis can occur between the learning that takes place in the clinical setting and that which occurs in the school of nursing. Figure 4.2 illustrates a cycle that can be used to integrate fully clinical experience with learning in the school or college.

The cycle illustrated in Figure 4.2 shows how clinical experience

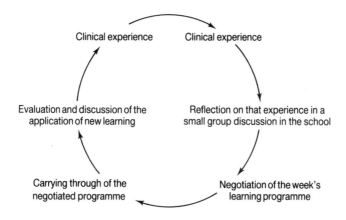

Figure 4.2   Integrating clinical and school learning

can be utilised and married up with school learning. When learners return to the school of nursing a discussion is held about their recent clinical experience. The tutor, acting as facilitator, then helps to draw out the new knowledge and skills that have been learned and the new knowledge and skills that *need* to be learned through further study or skills rehearsal. The tutor and learners then negotiate the week's programme by incorporating those learning needs into a timetable, which will also include those aspects of the prescribed syllabus as worked out by the school of nursing. This timetable is then worked through, via formal teaching sessions from tutors, student-led seminars, experiential learning workshops and so forth. Towards the end of the week the tutor and students evaluate their new learning and identify how that learning can be applied in the new clinical area.

It will be noted that this approach calls for flexibility and confidence on the part of the tutor and willingness to participate on the part of the learners. It will also be noted that the programme in the school of nursing is never predetermined before the learners return to the school. The only exceptions to this rule would be if outside speakers had to be booked in prior to the block. Such inclusions would be discussed with the learners and the rationale for including such speakers offered. This style of negotiated programme is completely in line with the adult learning (or andragogical) approach discussed in this book. This method also ensures that the *content* of the curriculum stays fresh and alive to the needs and wants of the learners and can incorporate changes in nursing as they occur. It is also a recipe for avoiding the development of 'dead knowledge' discussed above.

Learning in the clinical setting also needs careful monitoring to ensure that learners use that experience to the full. Two methods that can help are described in this book: the use of the journal and the mentor system. Both methods are student centred and allow for individual development.

An important issue in clinical learning is that it is *different* from learning in the school of nursing. Too often clinical areas try to set up 'ward classrooms' and qualified staff offer mini lectures in ward offices. This seems to indicate an important misunderstanding of the clinical learning process. Surely the basis of clinical learning should be the process of carrying out nursing with patients. The one thing that is always missing in the school of nursing and always present in the clinical setting is the presence of patients. Encounters with patients, whatever the clinical setting, should always form the basis of learning. It is notable that the experiential learning cycle described in Chapter 7 can be modified to encourage learning from clinical experience. Figure 4.3 offers a modified version of this cycle.

In this model of applied experiential learning theory the first stage is actual nursing experience. In stage two the learner, either as an

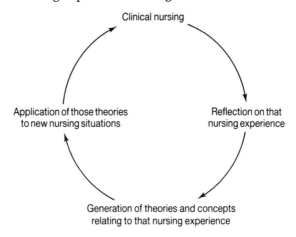

Figure 4.3 Learning from clinical experience

individual or as a member of a small clinical learning group, discusses that experience. From that experience she is encouraged to draw out theories and concepts that link her practice to the nursing literature and research. Out of that linking comes new direction for future nursing practice and that direction can be followed immediately in clinical nursing practice. In this model of learning the content of the 'clinical curriculum' always arises out of the individual nurse's nursing experience. Such a model has much to commend it in that the learning gained is necessarily and always grounded in human experience. If this clinical nursing model is linked to the school of nursing model offered above, learners should benefit from a nurse education that follows their own needs and wants, arises out of their everyday nursing experience and ensures that there is a constant link between what nursing researchers are finding, what the nursing literature has to say and what the nurse is actually experiencing in her everyday practice.

REFERENCES

Allan P and Jolley M (eds.) (1987) *The Curriculum in Nursing Education*. London: Croom Helm.

Blaney J (1974) Program development and curricula authority. In: *Program Development in Education*, eds. Blaney J, Housego I and McIntosh G. Vancouver: Centre for Continuing Education, University of British Columbia.

Brookfield S D (1986) *Understanding and Facilitating Adult Learning: A Comprehensive Analysis of Principles and Effective Practices*. Milton Keynes: Open University.

Burnard P (1987) Self and peer assessment. *Senior Nurse*, **6**(5): 17.

Burnard P (1989) Psychiatric nursing students' perceptions of experiential learning. *Nursing Times*, **85**(1): 52.

Davis B D (ed.) (1987) *Research into Nurse Education*. London: Croom Helm.

Freire P (1972) *Pedagogy of the Oppressed*. Harmondsworth: Penguin.

Greaves F (1987) *The Nursing Curriculum: Theory and Practice*. London: Croom Helm.

Henderson M S (ed.) (1982) *Nursing Education*. Edinburgh: Churchill Livingstone.

Jarvis P (1983) *Professional Education*. London: Croom Helm.

Kilty J (1981) *Self and Peer Assessment: A Collection of Papers*. Human Potential Research Project. Guildford, Surrey: University of Surrey.

Knowles M (1980) *The Modern Practice of Adult Education: From Pedagogy to Andragogy*, 2nd edn. Chicago: Follett.

Knowles M S and Associates (1984) *Andragogy in Action: Applying Modern Principles of Adult Learning*. California: Jossey Bass.

Lawton D (1973) *Social Change, Educational Theory and Curriculum Planning*. London: Hodder and Stoughton.

Maslow A (1972) *Motivation and Personality*, 2nd edn. New York: Harper and Row.

Melia K (1983) *Learning and Working*. London: Tavistock.

Nurses, Midwives and Health Visitors Rules Approval Order (1983) London: HMSO.

Peters R S (1966) *Ethics and Education*. London: Allen and Unwin.

Pirsig R (1974) *Zen and the Art of Motorcycle Maintenance*. London: Arrow.

Powell D (1982) *Learning to Relate?: A Study of Student Psychiatric Nurses' Views of their Preparation and Training*. London: RCN.

Rogers C R (1983) *Freedom to Learn for the Eighties*. Columbus, Ohio: Merrill.

CHAPTER 5

Deciding on Content

What should nurses' learn? Who decides? These are two central questions at the heart of curriculum planning. In attempting to answer those questions it may be useful to note four layers of decision-making that may be delineated:

1. The law relating to nurse education.
2. The UKCC/National Boards.
3. Directors of nurse education/senior tutors/tutors.
4. The students.

Any decisions that are made at a lower level on the above hierarchy will necessarily be dependent upon decisions at a higher level. It is worth working through the hierarchy to consider what effects the various decision-makers have on the content of nursing courses. It is interesting to consider this decision-making process in the light of the developments of nursing education as outlined in Part I of this book.

The Law Relating to Nurse Education

At the first level is the law relating to the content of nurse education. This is summarised in the Nurses, Midwives and Health Visitors Rules Approval Order (1983) (whose content was originally decided by the Statutory Bodies), which states that courses leading to qualification as a nurse must ensure that course members achieve the following competencies: they must be able to:

'● advise on the promotion of health and the prevention of illness;

- recognise situations that may be detrimental to the health and well-being of the individual;
- carry out those activities involved when conducting the comprehensive assessment of a person's nursing requirements;
- recognise the significance of the observations made and use these to develop an initial nursing assessment;
- devise a plan of nursing care based on the assessment with the co-operation of the patient, to the extent that this is possible, taking into account the medical prescription;
- implement the planned programme of nursing care and, where appropriate, teach and co-ordinate other members of the caring team who may be responsible for implementing specific aspects of the nursing care;
- review the effectiveness of the nursing care provided and, where appropriate, initiate any action that may be required;
- work in a team with other nurses, and with medical and para-medical staff and social workers;
- undertake the management of the care of a group of patients over a period of time and organise the appropriate support services related to the care of the particular type of patient with whom she is likely to come in contact when registered in that Part of the register for which the student intends to qualify.'

Considerable debate could be developed about the appropriateness or inappropriateness of these competencies; some nurses and nurse educators would no doubt wish to modify them or add to or subtract from them. The fact remains, however, that it is a nurse educator's duty to ensure that these competencies are met by students completing nurse training or education courses.

The UKCC/National Boards

Next, while the UKCC as the registering body has to define the form and content of an educational programme that is suitable for preparing nurses to be eligible for entry on to the Register, neither it nor the National Boards prescribe detailed content for any specific syllabus. This is somewhat different from the previous Statutory Bodies, such as the GNC, which produced comprehensive syllabi for the specific nursing disciplines (e.g. general nursing, psychiatry and mental handicap nursing). Instead, the National Boards approve courses produced by training institutions within the broad guidelines of the Nurses, Midwives and Health Visitors Rules and any other policy documents produced by the UKCC. It is interesting to note that the psychiatric nursing syllabus of 1982, which was the product of the GNC although published during the days of the 'shadow' UKCC and National Boards, went further than prescribing *content* and suggested also that experiential learning *methods* be used. As Kelly (1977) notes, syllabi more usually limit themselves to the prescription of knowledge and skills and leave decisions about teaching and learning to teachers.

Schools of Nursing

Each nursing school then has to *interpret* the guidelines laid down by the UKCC/National Boards according to their own educational philosophy and their own perception of their students' educational needs. This can lead to a rich diversity of approach to nursing education, curbed only by the fact of the National Boards' requirement for the individual local syllabus to be submitted to them for approval. This offers each school of nursing the opportunity to decide upon its own educational priorities, style of teaching and learning and methods of examination.

The specific choice of content for any particular course still remains with individual educators. Greaves (1987) offers the following guide to deciding upon content:

1. Knowledge of nursing or 'nursing knowledge' should include both theory and practice as inter-supporting elements of the activity of nursing.
2. Nursing knowledge should include information, concepts, skills and practices that are relevant, useful and capable of being known and learned in order to have direct utility value for the practice of nursing.
3. The knowledge included should be worthwhile and transferable to the nursing of patients.
4. The developed knowledge included in the curriculum has to have consensus in the sense that it needs to be agreed and acceptable and wherever possible based on the best available evidence.
5. The knowledge used in the curriculum should help to develop explanations or current practices, encourage critical analysis, influence problem-solving and help to establish in the students abilities to develop scientific approaches of enquiry.
6. The future preparation of nurse practitioners should be based on the use of knowledge through educational experiences that prepare the aspiring nurse for knowledge creation and innovative nursing practice.

Such guidelines do, of course, raise as many questions as they answer. A short list of such questions might be:

- What *are* the 'concepts, skills and practices that are relevant, useful and capable of being known and learned in order to have direct utility value for the practice of nursing'?
- What nursing knowledge is agreed as being worthwhile and transferable to the nursing of patients?
- Is there a consensus in the profession that nursing knowledge is agreed and based on the best available knowledge?
- Does the knowledge used in the curriculum enable the development of explanations, critical analysis and so forth? It is possible that nursing curricula in some schools of nursing are based on what Whitehead (1933) called 'dead knowledge': knowledge that is received and based more on tradition and established practice than on research and critical awareness.

Another way of considering how to make decisions about what content goes into a curriculum is to consider three domains of knowledge: propositional, practical and experiential. These are described and discussed in the next section. It is suggested that a balance of knowledge and skills from the three domains will make for a balanced curriculum regardless of whether that curriculum is prescribed by the school of nursing or negotiated with the learner group.

PROPOSITIONAL, PRACTICAL AND EXPERIENTIAL KNOWLEDGE

Propositional Knowledge

Propositional knowledge is that which is contained in theories or models. This includes the use of a model of nursing, which may be used as a framework to demonstrate the way in which the activity of nursing is viewed by the teachers and practitioners within a specific educational institution. This may be described as 'textbook' knowledge and is synonymous with Ryle's (1949) concept of 'knowing that', which is further developed in an educational context by Pring (1976). Thus a person may build up a considerable bank of facts, theories or ideas about a subject, person or thing without necessarily having any direct experience of that subject, person or thing. A person may, for example, develop a considerable propositional knowledge about midwifery without ever necessarily having been anywhere near a woman who is having a baby! Presumably it would be more useful to combine that knowledge with some practical experience but this does not necessarily have to be the case. This, then, is the domain of propositional knowledge. Obviously it is possible to have propositional knowledge about a great number of subject areas ranging from mathematics to literature or from counselling to social work. Any information contained in books must necessarily be of the propositional sort.

Practical Knowledge

Practical knowledge is knowledge that is developed through the acquisition of skills. Thus driving a car or giving an injection demonstrates practical knowledge although, equally, so does the use of counselling skills that involve specific verbal and non-verbal behaviours and intentional use of counselling interventions as described above. Practical knowledge is synonymous with Ryle's (1949) concept of 'knowing how', which was further developed, in an educational context, by Pring (1976). Usually more than mere 'knack', practical knowledge is the substance of a smooth performance of a practical or interpersonal skill. A considerable amount of a health professional's time is taken up with the demonstration of practical knowledge – often, but not always, of the interpersonal sort.

Traditionally, most educational programmes in schools and colleges have concerned themselves primarily with both propositional and practical knowledge, particularly the former. Thus the 'propositional knowledge' aspect of a person is the aspect that is often held in highest regard. Practical knowledge, although respected, is usually seen as slightly less important than the propositional sort. In this way the 'self' can become highly developed in one way – the propositional knowledge aspect – at the expense of being skilled in a practical sense.

Experiential Knowledge

The domain of experiential knowledge is knowledge gained through direct encounter with a subject, person or thing. It is the subjective and affective nature of that encounter that contributes to this sort of knowledge. Experiential knowledge is knowledge through relationship. Such knowledge is synonymous with

Rogers' (1983) description of experiential learning and with Polanyi's (1958) concepts of 'personal' and 'tacit' knowledge. If we reflect for a moment, we may discover that most of the things that are really important to us belong in this domain. If, for example, we consider our personal relationships with other people, we discover that what we like or love about them cannot be reduced to a series of propositional statements, yet the feelings we have for them are vital and part of what is most important in our lives. Most encounters with others contain the possible seeds of experiential knowledge. It is only when we are so detached from other people that we treat them as objects that no experiential learning can occur.

Not all experiential knowledge is tied exclusively to relationships with other people. For example, I had considerable propositional knowledge about America before I went there. When I went there all that propositional knowledge was changed considerably. What I had known was changed by my direct experience of the country. I had developed *experiential* knowledge of the place. Experiential knowledge is not of the same type or order as propositional or practical knowledge. It is, nevertheless, important knowledge in that it affects everything else we think about or do.

Experiential knowledge is necessarily personal and idiosyncratic. Indeed, as Rogers (1985) points out, it may be difficult to convey to another person in words. Words tend to be loaded with personal (often experiential) meanings and thus to understand each other we need to understand the nature of the way in which the people with whom we converse use words. It is arguable, however, that such experiential knowledge is sometimes conveyed to others through gesture, eye contact, tone of voice, inflection and all the other non-verbal and paralinguistic aspects of communication (Argyle, 1975). Indeed, it may be experiential knowledge that is passed on when two people (for example a nurse and her client) become very involved with each other in a conversation, a learning encounter or counselling.

A Balance of Knowledge

It is suggested that a balance between propositional, practical and experiential knowledge may make for a varied and appropriate content for a nursing course. Examples of propositional, practical and experiential knowledge in the field of nursing are offered below. It will be noted that the sorts of knowledge that are contained in the domains of propositional and practical knowledge are far more in keeping with the content of a traditional nursing curriculum. Arguably, the addition of experiential knowledge adds the personal and 'human' element that enables the learner to place herself, with all her experiences, feelings, beliefs and values, within the context of the job that she does.

Examples of Propositional Knowledge in a Nursing Curriculum
- Nursing models.
- Ethics.
- Research theory.
- Medicine.
- Psychiatry.

Examples of Practical Knowledge in a Nursing Curriculum
- How to give an injection.
- How to break bad news.
- How to communicate clearly on the telephone.
- How to do a wound dressing.

Examples of Experiential Knowledge in a Nursing Curriculum
- Personal feelings.
- Personal beliefs.
- Prejudices.
- Strengths and weaknesses.
- Hidden emotions.

In summary and in closing the discussion on the incorporation of the three domains of knowledge into the nursing curriculum, it is worth noting Skillbeck's (in Jenkins and Shipman, 1976) suggestions that subject matter in any curriculum be all of the following:

'1. Rational, coherent and fundamental – ordered and organised to a framework of rules, principles and basic ideas; capable of being systematically related to other themes, topics and bodies of knowledge; rich in the powers of explanation, criticism and problem solving; able to stand up to relevant tests of validity and reliability.
2. Contemporary – true according to current knowledge and theories; relatable to contemporary problems and issues.
3. Socially relevant – having wide and varied application to society, its needs and issues.
4. Action oriented – so selected and designed as to enable learners to undertake tasks, confront problems and achieve intellectual and practical competencies.

5. Broad and balanced.
6. Learnable and teachable – having a structure and sequence which fit the needs and capabilities of teachers and learners.
7. Intrinsically interesting and meaningful.'

Skillbeck's criteria offer all the characteristics that should characterise a useful and satisfying nursing curriculum: variety, current relevance, social applicability, action, breadth and depth, practicality and interest.

PUTTING THE SYLLABUS INTO ACTION

Once a school of nursing has had approval for its syllabus it may then proceed to put the syllabus into action. It is at this point that tutors and learners can negotiate certain aspects of the course. The question here must be: what is left to negotiate? If there are legal requirements for nursing education, which are approved by the National Boards when written into course programmes, it would seem that little is left for negotiation.

There are at least two issues here. One is the degree of flexibility and room for negotiation that a school of nursing builds into its proposals to the National Board. It is possible, for example, for a school to justify an educational philosophy along the lines of student-centred or adult learning principles and to write these into the submission documents. In this way a mandate is obtained from the National Board to move further into student negotiation. On the other hand, there may be a limit to the degree of flexibility that will be accepted by the National Boards. There is a danger that the people who become officers or nurse advisors at the National Boards will slip behind current thinking on education in comparison with the tutors and course organisers (who may be in the process of obtaining degrees or higher degrees in educational topics). This slipping back may also be combined with a tendency for established bureaucratic structures to veer on the side of safety. The net result may be viewed in two ways. On the one hand, the process of having the National Boards as boards of approval can ensure that adequate checks and balances are incorporated into the system. On the other hand, the whole process may be seen as reactionary and stifling. Either way, this is one path towards working on negotiation of content – by writing negotiation into the curriculum proposal.

The second method of initiating negotiation is for the curriculum submission to concern itself mostly with *content* and thus to leave decisions about *method* to individual tutors and their students. In a sense this is what teachers and students have always done: teachers have normally been free to decide on the best way to encourage the learning of a particular topic by a particular group of students. It is here that an interesting paradox arises out of the psychiatric nursing syllabus of 1982. As noted above, that syllabus suggested that experiential learning methods should be widely used. In making this prescription the syllabus could be seen to restrict tutor and student negotiation, for if the prescribed method of learning is experiential, other methods of teaching and learning are necessarily ruled out. It may be argued, therefore, that a syllabus is most useful when it serves as a framework of content to be covered in a course and nothing else.

It is also worth noting at this point that a distinction is often made between a model of the curriculum based on *content* and a model based on *process* (Stenhouse, 1975; Wells, 1987). Content is fairly straightforward and refers to the subject matter of a curriculum, as discussed above. Process, referred to here, is concerned with how learners learn and how knowledge and skills are developed. Some nurse educators feel that nurse education should be more concerned with process than with content. A moment's reflection, however, will reveal that there can be no such thing as a curriculum without content, nor can there be a curriculum that is mostly concerned with process. If a curriculum concerned itself mostly with process, what would be learned? Whatever specific answer is offered to the question, undoubtedly *something* would be learned – this 'something' would be content.

To avoid the content question or to assume that learners can automatically identify their own content is naive. No learner coming to a course can be expected to know what it is he wants or needs to learn in order to enter a profession. Not to identify a framework of content is to omit an important aspect of curriculum design. Arguably, those who would argue for a 'process' model of the curriculum inevitably have some 'content' lined up in the form of a 'hidden agenda'. In other words, they would claim not to influence the content of a course in a particular direction but by their words, arguments, contributions to the group and a thousand other ways, would subtly (and sometimes not so subtly) lead the learners in a particular direction. Far better, perhaps, to make the 'content' aspect of a curriculum explicit in the first place. Whether or not that declaration of content is spelt out in behavioural objectives, expressive objectives or outcomes is probably not so important. Educational theory and practice is not yet a precise science; the way in which objectives or outcomes are couched is not yet as critical as some would have us believe.

Another point may be made about what is left to negotiate in terms of content. The Nurses, Midwives and Health Visitors Rules and advice from the National Boards offer an *outline* of the knowledge and skills that must be included in a training/education course for nurses. Such rules and syllabi still leave room for individual and group learning needs. While no course ever includes everything that is contained in a syllabus, neither need any course forget that different students and different groups have different learning needs. It is notable, too, that teachers are nearly always 'teaching in private'; what they do or say in the classroom is rarely monitored by senior staff. In this sense, they have considerable autonomy and flexibility over how they interpret any given syllabus.

Negotiating Aspects of Content

What considerations need to be borne in mind and when negotiating aspects of the content of a nursing course? A model drawn from the management literature may help here. Adair (1988) offers a simple model of three aspects of management (Figure 5.1). The model may be used to help to identify how to negotiate the content of a curriculum for a particular group and/or particular school.

Task Needs
In terms of a nursing course the task needs of a given group can be identified fairly easily. They include at least the following:

- Learning the specific knowledge and skills required to become a nurse.
- Learning sufficient to be successful in assessments and examinations.
- Offering educational and interpersonal support to each other.

Generally these task needs may be derived from the Nurses, Midwives and Health Visitors Rules and the syllabi discussed above. In a sense all learners in all schools of nursing face a similar set of task needs: the fact that learners are on a particular course leading to a particular professional qualification makes this true.

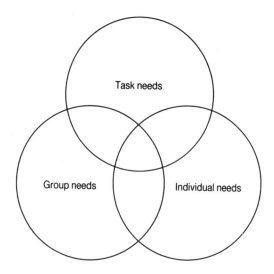

Figure 5.1 Model of group needs (after Adair, 1988)

Group Needs

Separate from, yet related to, task needs are the needs of the specific group. As already noted, students do not come to nurse education as 'blank slates'. They come as people from varied backgrounds with varying degrees of knowledge and experience. It is when they become a group that all their past knowledge and experience becomes a resource for the group. A number of things follow from these issues. First, not all the group members will require the same sort of thing from the course. Second, some group members will be able to learn from other members, and third, if the group is to stay together, some *individual* needs will have to be suppressed in order for the group to remain intact. Group membership always involves a degree of conflict between the needs of individuals and the needs of 'the group'. Careful planning can ensure that the needs of the group, in terms of the content of a course, are catered for. While the national requirements can help to some degree, there is also a requirement for tutors to be open to the specific needs of a particular group.

Individual Needs

As noted in the previous paragraph, groups are made up of individuals who have particular needs above and beyond both the task needs and the group needs. Nurse training and education can also take account of particular interests, needs and wants of individual students. This may mean that the learner is offered tutorials with a personal tutor or that individual project work is encouraged in order to facilitate idiosyncratic learning requirements. Just because learners are members of a group of other learners does not mean that they always have to work together as a single unit. Individual learning contracts are one way of encouraging people to study the areas that are of particular interest to them.

The point of the model outlined in Figure 5.1 above is that it should encourage a sense of balance between the three aspects of management. If any one aspect becomes overdeveloped, that overdevelopment is at the expense of group and educational harmony.

This chapter has considered some of the influences and constraints on the aspect of curriculum that is concerned with content. As we have seen, the issue of content is a complex one that involves the interplay of legal issues, the approval of National Boards and more local philosophies, combined with individual learning needs, all of which must combine to produce a nurse who is eligible to be entered on the UKCC's Register.

REFERENCES

Adair J (1988) *Effective Leadership: A Modern Guide to Developing Leadership Skills*. London: Pan.
Argyle M (1975) *The Psychology of Interpersonal Behaviour*. Harmondsworth: Penguin.
Greaves F (1987) *The Nursing Curriculum: Theory and Practice*. London: Croom Helm.
Jenkins D and Shipman M D (1976) *Curriculum: An Introduction*. London: Basic Books.
Kelly V A (1977) *The Curriculum*. London: Harper and Row.
Nurses, Midwives and Health Visitors Rules Approval Order (1983). London: HMSO.
Polanyi M (1958) *Personal Knowledge*. Chicago: University of Chicago Press.
Pring R (1976) *Knowledge and Schooling*. London: Basic Books.
Rogers C R (1983) *Freedom to Learn for the Eighties*. Columbus, Ohio: Merrill.
Rogers C R (1985) Towards a more human science of the person. *Journal of Humanistic Psychology*, **25**(4): 7–24.
Ryle G (1949) *The Concept of Mind*. Harmondsworth: Peregrine.

Stenhouse L (1975) *An Introduction to Curriculum Research and Development.* London: Heinemann.

Wells J (1987) Curriculum evaluation. In: *The Curriculum in Nursing Education,* P Allan and M Jolley (eds.). London: Croom Helm.

Whitehead A N (1933) *The Aims of Education.* London: Benn.

CHAPTER 6

Student-centred Learning

FACILITATION OR TEACHING?

The accent in nursing education is towards the educational encounter being student-centred rather than teacher-centred, and appropriately adult-centred. In this approach the aim is not to initiate the group participants into particular ways of knowing, as Peters (1969) would argue, but to encourage those people to think about their own experience and to transform their personal knowledge and skills through the processes of reflection, discussion and action. In the student-centred approach to learning, the nurse educator acts as a *facilitator of learning* rather than as a *teacher*.

The notion of 'teacher' suggests one who passes on knowledge to others, who instructs and manages learning for others. The notion of facilitation has other connotations and these are developed in this chapter alongside the practical issues that need to be addressed if the nurse educator is to function as a facilitator.

King (1984) offers the following suggestions about the nature of the facilitator's role:

- Facilitators must believe that students should make their own decisions and think for themselves.
- They must refrain from assuming an authoritative role and should adopt a more facilitative and listening position.
- They must accept diversity of race, sex, values, etc. among their students.
- They must be willing to accept all viewpoints unconditionally and not impose their personal values on the students. The ability to entertain alternatives and to negotiate no-lose sol-

utions to problems often leads to group decisions that are more beneficial for both the individual and the group.

Certain stages in the facilitation process can be described and the facilitator needs to be aware of the processes that can occur in groups. The stages described here are modified from those offered by Knowles (1975) in his discussion of facilitating learning groups for adults.

It is arguable that facilitation of learning has more in common with group therapy than it does with teaching. It is recommended that the person who sets out to become a group facilitator gain experience as a member of a number of different sorts of group before leading one himself. In this way he will not only learn about group processes experientially but will also see a number of facilitator styles. As Heron (1977a) points out, in the early stages of becoming a facilitator it is often helpful to base your style on a facilitator that you have seen in action. Later, the style becomes modified in the light of your own experience and you develop your own approach.

Stages in the Facilitation Process

Setting the Learning Climate
The first aspect of helping adults to learn is the creation of an atmosphere in which adult learners feel comfortable and thus able to learn. This is particularly important when it comes to developing interpersonal skills through experiential learning. Unlike more formal classroom learning, the student-centred approach asks of the learners that they try things out, take some risks and experiment. If this is to happen at all, it needs to be undertaken in an atmosphere of mutual trust and understanding.

The first aspect of the setting of a learning climate is to ensure that the environment is appropriate. Rows of desks and chairs are reminiscent of earlier schooldays. For the adult nursing learning group it is often better and certainly more egalitarian if learners and facilitator sit together in a closed circle of chairs.

In the early stages of a learning group it is useful too if the group members spend time getting to know each other. 'Icebreakers' are sometimes used for this purpose. An icebreaker is a simple group activity that is designed to relax people and allow them to 'let their hair down' a little, thus creating a more relaxed atmosphere, arguably more conducive to learning. An example of an icebreaker is as follows:

> The group stands up and group members mill around the room at will. At a signal from the facilitator, each person stops and introduces herself to the nearest person and shares some personal details. Then each person moves on and at a further signal, stops and greets another person in a similar way. This series of millings and pairings can continue until each group member has met all the others including the facilitator.

Other examples of icebreaking activities can be found elsewhere (Heron, 1973; Burnard, 1985). Their aim is to produce a relaxed atmosphere in which learning can take place, and a further gain is that they encourage group participation and the learning of names. They are used by many facilitators in the experiential learning field. Some people, however (including the author) feel more comfortable with a more straightforward form of introduction. The argument here is that learners coming to a new learning experience are already apprehensive. Many carry with them memories of past learning experiences, which may or may not have been of the 'formal' sort. To introduce those people to icebreakers too early may be to alienate them before they start. The icebreaker, by its very unorthodoxy, may surprise and upset them. A simpler form of introductory activity is to invite each person in turn to tell the rest of the group the following information:

- her name;
- where she works and her position in the team or organisation;
- a few details about herself that are nothing to do with work.

It is helpful if the facilitator sets the pace for the activity by first introducing herself in this way. A precedent is thus set and the group members have some idea of both what to say and how much to say. The author recalls forgetting this principle when running a learning session in the Netherlands. As a result, each group member talked for about ten minutes and what was intended to be a short introductory activity turned into a lengthy exercise! The golden rule, perhaps, is keep the activity short and sharp and keep the atmosphere 'light' and easy going.

Once group members have begun to get to know each other, either through the use of icebreakers or by the introductory activity described above, the facilitator should deal with 'domestic' issues regarding the group's life. These will include the following:

- When the group will break for refreshments and meal breaks and when it will end.
- A discussion of the aims of the group.
- A discussion of the 'voluntary principle': that learners should decide for themselves whether or not they will take part in any given activity suggested by the facilitator, and that no-one should feel pressurised, either by the facilitator or by the power of group pressure, into taking part in any activity. It is worth pointing out that if a person finds herself to be the only person sitting out on a particular activity, she should not feel under any further obligation either to take part or to justify her decision not to take part.
- Issues relating to smoking in the group when smokers are present.
- Any other issues identified by either the facilitator or by group members.

This early discussion of group 'rules' is an important part of the process of setting the learning climate. The structure engendered by this part of the day helps to allow everyone to feel part of the decision-making and learning process.

Identifying Learning Resources
In this stage both learners and tutor identify the resources for learning that are present within the group. This may be done with the aid of 'needs/offers' board. A large flip-chart sheet or area of a black or white board is divided into two columns: 'needs' and 'offers'. Learners and tutors then fill this chart in appropriately at the beginning of a course or block of learning. Clearly, this approach cannot be used at the start of the *first* such course or block, where neither tutors nor learners will know each other's skills and knowledge bases. After an introductory programme, however, the needs/offers board can be used to help determine the content of all future learning encounters.

Once both tutors and learners have written down their learning needs and what they have to offer the group, each member of the group is then encouraged to put a tick against the items that they feel will most usefully be included in the learning period. Figure 6.1 illustrates a completed board and one that can then be used to timetable the course, block or week.

This approach to identifying needs and resources can be used for

Needs	Offers
• More on the nervous system	• Seminar on anxiety
• Revision of drugs	• Overview of sociology
• More on counselling skills	• Care of the dying person
• Orem's model of nursing	• Counselling activities
• Using the nursing process	• Research skills seminar
• Relaxation activities	• Stress workshop
• Review of digestive system	• Applying models
• More on care of the elderly	• Visit to probation office (2 days' notice required)
• Revision of basic dressing techniques	• Lecture on drug abuse
• Medical nursing revision	• Handling aggression

Figure 6.1 Example of a completed needs/offers board

1-day workshops as well as for week-long study perio ls. It depends for its success on all members of the learning group being committed to full negotiation of content. Having said that, it would seem reasonable that the tutor retains the right to add certain 'compulsory' topics to any given programme in line with her perception of what is required to fulfil a particular syllabus.

Planning the Learning Encounter. Once the learning group's needs and resources have been identified, the group can draw up a learning contract. Types of contract can range from the informally agreed list of topics that will be used as the basis of discussion and learning during the day or week, to a planned identification of what will be learned, how it will be learned and how learning will be evaluated. Figure 6.2 offers one example of the more formally drawn up type of contract. Such a contract will draw from

Topic	Time	Method	Evaluation
Day 1			
1. Review of nervous system	1.00–3.00	Tutor-led discussion	Verbal
2. Discussion of counselling skills	3.30–4.30	Student-led discussion	None
Day 2			
1. Practice of counselling skills	9.00–12.30	Micro-skills teaching by tutor	Demo.
2. Using Orem's model in practice	1.00–4.30	Student-led seminars	Test
If required, the topic headings can be turned into learning objectives			

Figure 6.2 Example of part of a group learning contract

the following elements:

- Non-negotiable content drawn from the syllabus.
- Wants and offers.

The non-negotiable content drawn from the syllabus may serve as a theme for the learning period. On the other hand, it is important that the content drawn from the needs and offers lists are not seen as 'additions' to an already worked out timetable. The aim is not to offer learners concessions but to negotiate fully a timetable that best suits their wants and needs, yet which also fully prepares them for any examinations and practical work that they will face. The tutor who facilitates the drawing up of this initial learning contract will need to exercise considerable tact and diplomacy in handling the tension between individual and group needs on the one hand and the requirements of the syllabus on the other.

An alternative approach to using group learning contracts is for each learner to draw up one for her own use. This may mean that a given group of students does not meet together for the entire period of learning but that some students will be working on their own while others are attending lectures, seminars, discussions and practical learning sessions.

Running the Learning Group. All that remains is for the learning session to progress along the lines that have been negotiated with the group. The facilitator's task is to ensure the smooth running of the group. Variety of method is an important consideration in ensuring that all members get what they need from the learning encounter, and the following is a short list of methods that may be used:

- Lectures.
- Tutor-led seminars.
- Student-led seminars.
- Tutor-led discussions.
- Student-led discussions.
- Leaderless discussions.
- Experiential learning activities (see Chapters 7 and 8).
- Buzz groups (small, short discussion groups to generate ideas or solutions).
- Individual learning sessions.
- Demonstrations.
- Visits.
- Invited speakers.

- Small group project work.
- Small group discussions followed by large group plenary sessions.

It is probably fair to say that most tutors will be armed with a variety of teaching and learning strategies (but will probably only use a limited number of them), while many learners coming to student-centred learning for the first time will tend to imagine that 'teaching and learning' necessarily involves having someone at the front of the group who leads it and does most of the talking. It is helpful if all learners coming to student-centred learning from more traditional approaches are offered a number of sessions on:

- the philosophy of student-centred learning and a rationale for its use;
- the range of teaching/learning methods that is available;
- practice in a range of teaching/learning methods and feedback on their use.

If student-centred learning is to succeed, it must involve the learners in every respect, including the skilful use of teaching and learning methods. Learning to use these methods is never wasted for they can be used again and again in future learning encounters, both within educational establishments and within the clinical setting. In the clinical area it is clearly inappropriate to use a formal 'lecture' method. It is not uncommon, however, to find mini-classrooms set up in wards and departments that exactly mimic the sorts of traditional learning approaches that the nurses working there have been subject to. The student-centred approach to learning can encourage the appropriate use of appropriate learning aids.

Closing the Group
Each facilitator will probably develop her own style of closing the group at the end of the day or at the end of a workshop. A traditional way is through a summary of what the day has been about. There is an important limitation in this method, which aims at 'closure'. It is asserted that while the facilitator is summing up in this way, she is doing two things that are not particularly helpful. First, she is putting into her own words those of the group members. Second, while she is 'closing' in this way group members are often, silently, closing off their thoughts about the day or the workshop in much the same way that schoolchildren begin to put their books away as soon as a teacher sums up at the

end of a lesson. It may be far better to leave the session open-ended and to avoid any sort of summing up. Alternatively, rather than allowing the day or the workshop to end rather abruptly, the facilitator may choose to use one or more of the following closing and evaluating activities.

Closing Activity 1. Each person in turn makes a short statement about what she liked *least* about the day or about the workshop. Each person in turn then makes a short statement about what she liked *most* about the day or the workshop. No-one has to justify what she says for her statement is taken as a personal evaluation of her feelings and experience.

Closing Activity 2. Each person in turn makes a short statement about three things that she feels she has learned during the day or the workshop. This may or may not be followed by a discussion on the day's learning.

Closing Activity 3. The group has an 'unfinished business' session. Group members are encouraged to share any comments, either of a positive or negative nature, that they may have about the day or the workshop. The rationale for this activity is that such sharing helps to avoid bottled-up feelings and increases a sense of group cohesion.

These, then, are the stages of a typical student-centred learning session and they may be adapted to suit the particular needs of the group and facilitator. The final part of the learning encounter may also involve checking through the group's learning contract to see whether or not various aspects have been covered in sufficient depth and whether or not changes need to be made to that contract.

FACILITATOR STYLE

Each facilitator needs to make decisions about what to do when working with a particular learning group. What she does in the group may be called her style. Clearly, facilitator styles will vary from person to person according to a number of variables, including previous group experience, teacher training, knowledge and skill levels, personal preferences, personal value systems and personal beliefs about the nature of education. However, it is useful if the facilitator of learning (and particularly the one who is new to facilitation) can consider what decisions she needs to make about her style *prior* to engaging in facilitation. Heron (1977b) suggests six dimensions of facilitator style that can help in such decision-making. These are:

'Directive....................Non-directive
Interpretative ....Non-interpretative
Confronting..............Non-confronting
Cathartic ....Non-cathartic
Structuring ....Un-structuring
Disclosing.................Non-disclosing'

The tutor who uses the directive–non-directive dimension will make decisions about how much she intervenes in the process of development of the group. At one end of the dimension the tutor may decide to control group discussion almost completely by asking questions of the group and also by maintaining overall control of what happens in the group. At the other end of the dimension the tutor will play a role that is lower in profile and will maintain little or no control over what happens in the group, preferring the learners to decide on the way in which the group develops. While the non-directive end of the dimension is more student-centred, there are clearly times when tutor intervention will enable the group to move on and develop further. The skilled facilitator is probably one who can make appropriate decisions about when to be directive and when to remain in the background.

The interpretative–non-interpretative dimension is concerned with the degree to which the tutor does or does not offer explanations for what happens in the group. Interpretations of group processes can be made from a number of different points of view, including, at least, the following: psychodynamic, sociological, transactional analytical, transpersonal and political. The tutor who chooses to use interpretation in order to help the learners make sense of what is happening in the group offers a theoretical framework for the learners to work with. The tutor who offers no interpretation allows the learners to make their own decisions about what is happening and allows them to construct and develop their own theories. The only problem facing the tutor who never uses an interpretative style of group leadership is that she may have to acknowledge that some groups will neither notice group processes developing nor construct theories to account for what happens.

The next dimension is concerned with the degree to which the tutor does or does not confront the group at any given time in the group's development. At one end of the dimension the tutor is very challenging and draws attention to illogicalities and inconsistencies in group arguments. At the other end of the dimension she sits back and allows members of the group to challenge group debate. Again, as with the other dimensions, it is probably useful if the facilitator can learn to be appropriately confronting or appropriately passive according to circumstances.

The cathartic–non-cathartic dimension refers to the amount of emotional release that the facilitator allows or seeks in a learning group. It is arguable that during the process of learning counselling and group skills it is helpful if group participants are allowed to express their feelings as part of the experiential learning process. Sometimes, too, arguments and discussions can be sharpened if participants are allowed to express strong feelings. At other times, however, it is more appropriate that emotional release does not become part of the group process. In a clinical teaching session, for example, or during a ward round, it may not be appropriate for learners to express their feelings directly. It may be more appropriate if that emotion is expressed later during a student–tutor discussion.

There are specific skills involved in helping people to express emotion. Heron (1977c) argues that in the UK we have developed a 'non-cathartic society', in which the general norm is to bottle up rather than express emotion. He suggests various methods for helping groups to release pent-up emotion, and courses in developing cathartic skills are frequently offered by colleges and extramural departments of universities.

Emotional release is part of the human condition. It is also frequently a part of the experience of being a patient. If learners *never* have the opportunity to explore their own feelings, then, arguably, they will be less well prepared for handling the emotional release of their patients. This is not to advocate frequent therapy or encounter groups as part of the educational experience but to acknowledge the need for tutors to consider the inclusion of the development of cathartic skills at some points in the nurse education programme.

The structuring–un-structuring dimension is a vital one in terms of student-centred nurse education. The highly structuring tutor will organise the timetable, decide upon content, carry through the lessons and evaluate the whole procedure. In other words, the *structuring* facilitator is not particularly student-centred. On the other hand, the facilitator who is totally un-structuring may be one whose learning sessions are an educational 'free for all', with little coherence or development. Again, the answer seems to lie in a sense of balance and an ability to decide when to offer structure to a group and when to allow the group to develop its own.

Heron's final dimension is the disclosing–non-disclosing one. The disclosing facilitator is one who shares with learners much of her own thoughts and feelings as they emerge. In this sense she becomes a fellow traveller of the learners. In 1964 Jourard suggested that 'disclosure begets disclosure'. It seems likely that the tutor who is able to share something of herself with her learners is more likely to encourage them to share something of themselves with the group. Thus the process of education becomes a humanising process.

On the other hand, there are times when non-disclosure is appropriate. If the tutor is *too* disclosing, she may find that she inhibits group participants. Most of us have experienced the person who, at the drop of a hat, tells us his life story or who too readily discloses his own thoughts or feelings. Almost as important as *whether or not* we disclose to a group is the decision about *when* we disclose. As with most things in life, timing is of the utmost importance. Sometimes to hold back and keep our thoughts and feelings to ourselves can encourage quieter members of the group to develop the courage to disclose.

The six dimensions of facilitator style have wide application across many different sorts of learning group. Tutors may use them in seminar groups, in organising discussions, in running support groups and in running learning groups in clinical settings. The dimensions may also be offered to learners as a framework for considering their own decisions about running groups. Whenever we engage in a learning encounter we make certain decisions about how to proceed. The dimensions of facilitator style offered here allow for clear-cut *prior* decisions to be made. They also allow for 'fine tuning' while the group is in progress. The person who has internalised and understood the range of possibilities contained within the six dimensions can quickly change tack while working within a group, yet do that with some precision.

REFERENCES

Brandes D and Phillips R (1984) *The Gamester's Handbook*, Vol. 2. London: Hutchinson.

Burnard P (1985) *Learning Human Skills: A Guide for Nurses*. London: Heinemann.

Heron J (1973) *Experiential Training Techniques*. Human Potential Research Project. Guildford, Surrey: University of Surrey.

Heron J (1977a) *Behaviour Analysis in Education and Training*. Human Potential Research Project. Guildford, Surrey: University of Surrey.

Heron J (1977b) *Dimensions of Facilitator Style*. Human Potential Research Project. Guildford, Surrey: University of Surrey.

Jourard S (1964) *The Transparent Self*. New Jersey: Van Nostrand.

King E C (1984) *Affective Education in Nursing: A Guide to Teaching and Assessment*. Maryland: Aspen.

Knowles M (1975) *Self-Directed Learning*. New York: Cambridge.

Peters R S (1969) *The Ethics of Education*. London: Allen and Unwin.

CHAPTER 7

Experiential Learning

Experiential learning has become a frequent subject of discussion in schools of nursing and in the literature (Bailey, 1983; McNulty, 1984; Burnard, 1985; Miles, 1987). The 1982 syllabus of training for psychiatric nursing students recommended that such methods be used in the development of interpersonal skills in student nurse training. This chapter briefly explores the concept of experiential learning by defining it, identifying some experiential learning methods and exploring two of those methods in some detail.

EXPERIENTIAL LEARNING DEFINED

Experiential learning can be defined as learning through doing. However, it is also more than that. It is learning through *reflecting on doing*. In all aspects of our actions we have at least two choices: just to act or to *notice* how we act. It is only through noticing what it is that we do that we can hope to learn about ourselves and our behaviour. To 'just act' is to act blindly, unawarely. This is what happens when we do not learn from experience. In a sense, it is as simple as that: if we are to learn from what we do, we must notice what we do and reflect on it. To notice what we do is to allow ourselves to evaluate action and to choose the next piece of behaviour. This is living in a more precise way. Now, clearly we cannot notice our behaviour and actions all the time. But in terms of the relationships we have with our clients we owe it to them to notice our behaviour more frequently than we may be doing at present. To do this noticing is to engage in what Heron (1973) calls 'conscious use of the self': using behaviour and the self in a conscious, therapeutic manner. To make conscious use of the self during interpersonal relationships is to enhance the likeliness of our relationships being therapeutic.

Two examples from practice may help here. First, Andrew Jones, a charge nurse, is having problems at home. As a result he unthinkingly looks unapproachable to his patients. He frowns a lot and has a tendency to be rather abrupt with them. Thus his patients find it more and more difficult to talk to him and tend to keep their conversations with him to a minimum. He continues to be unaware of the effect that he is having on them because he remains distracted by his own problems.

Sarah Davies, on the other hand, is a ward sister who is also having domestic and marital problems. She, however, makes a conscious effort to leave those problems behind her when she goes to work. She also pays attention to how she presents herself to her colleagues and her patients, both in the way she dresses for work and also with regard to her 'body language'. She has learned to notice, to reflect on her behaviour and to make conscious use of self. As a result her patients feel better from talking to her and find her approachable. This positive effect on her patients also makes *her* feel better and makes it a little easier for her to face the domestic problems that she picks up again when she returns home.

There is a second sense of the term 'experiential learning'. We all learn through experience, whether directly through taking action, through being involved in a situation or by observing others. In this sense every situation is an experiential learning situation. To describe experiential learning in such broad terms would be rather fruitless, however, as it would make the concept so huge as to render it unmanageable. To make things a little more clear, we may identify three aspects of experiential learning:

1. Personal experience.
2. Reflection on that experience.
3. The transformation of knowledge and meaning as a result of that reflection.

A fourth stage, in which we *use* what we have learned, may also be added to the first three and thus a continuous cycle of experience–reflection–transformation of knowledge and meaning–action/experience is created (Figure 7.1).

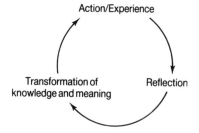

Figure 7.1   An experiential learning cycle

EXAMPLES OF EXPERIENTIAL LEARNING IN NURSING

All nurses learn through reflecting on their practice. Experiential learning does not occur, as we have noted, when we do not reflect on our practice. The issue of reflection is a crucial one. In order to learn we must first notice or as the mystic Ousepensky (1988) put it, we must learn to *remember ourselves*. Ousepensky argues that for much of our lives we are only half conscious or we are working on 'automatic pilot'. When we do this, we no longer register what is happening to us. Indeed, Ousepensky argues that if we do not remember ourselves and notice what is happening to us, we will not commit to memory the events that are taking place within and around us. Instead, we must learn to cultivate an increasing awareness of our senses and of our changing thoughts, feelings and actions. Examples of how this reflective ability can help us to learn in nursing are given below. A reflective ability can help us in:

- Learning through talking to clients.
- Working in the field.
- Reflecting on past clinical experiences.
- Comparing notes with other health-care professionals.
- Noticing personal thoughts, feelings and emotions.
- Exploring feelings in small groups.
- Attendance at experiential learning workshops.
- Learning counselling and group therapy by working with clients.
- Keeping journals and diaries.
- Receiving positive and negative feedback from colleagues and peers.

- Comparing past and present situations.
- Using relaxation and meditational activities.
- Consciously managing time.
- Using problem-solving devices and strategies.
- Entering into personal therapy/counselling.
- Consciously trying new coping strategies.
- Learning by 'sitting with Nellie': learning on the job.
- Trial and error learning.
- Learning by experimentation.
- Reading about, then trying out, new ideas.
- Consciously changing role.
- Practising new interpersonal skills.
- Learning group facilitation by running groups.

THE HISTORICAL DEVELOPMENT OF EXPERIENTIAL LEARNING

Clearly, people have always learned from experience. However, the idea of experiential learning as an educational concept is a relatively recent one. It will be useful to review some of the historical roots of the concept in order to make sense of some of the experiential learning methods that follow in the next chapter.

Drawing on the work of American pragmatic philosopher John Dewey (1916, 1938), Keeton et al (1976) describe experiential learning as including learning through the process of living and include work experience, skills developed through hobbies and interests and non-formal educational activities. This approach to definition is reflected in the FEU project report *Curriculum Opportunity*, which asserts that, for the purposes of that report, experiential learning refers to the knowledge and skills acquired through life and work experience and study (FEU, 1983).

Pfeiffer and Goodstein (1982) offer a different approach to the concept by describing an 'experiential learning cycle', which spells out the possible *process* of experiential learning (Figure 7.2). This cycle not only suggests the format for organising experiential learning but also makes tacit reference to the way in which people learn through experience.

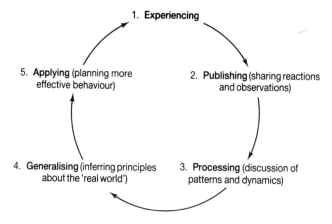

Figure 7.2 Experiential learning cycle (after Pfeiffer and Goodstein, 1982)

Kolb (1984) was more explicit about this learning process in his experiential learning model (Figure 7.3). In this model concrete experience is the starting point for a reflective process that echoes Freire's (1972) concept of 'praxis'. Praxis, for Freire, is the combination of reflection and action-on-the-world: a transforming process that is one of man's distinguishing features and one that enables him to change his view of the world and, ultimately, to change the world itself.

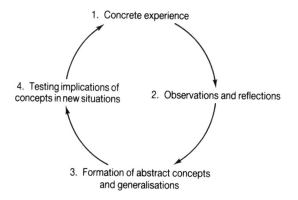

Figure 7.3 Experiential learning model (after Kolb, 1984)

Malcolm Knowles (1980), the American adult educator, took a different approach to the definition of experiential learning. He described the activities that took place within the concept and thus listed the following, which he called 'participatory experiential techniques':

'Group discussion, cases, critical incidents, simulations, role-play, skills practice exercises, field projects, action projects, laboratory methods, consultative supervision (coaching), demonstrations, seminars, work conferences, counselling, group therapy and community development.'

His list seems so all-inclusive that he seems to have been saying that experiential learning techniques were any techniques other than the lecture method or private, individual study, and that experiential learning was synonymous with participant and discovery learning. Boydell (1976) took just such a position when he asserted that:

'Experiential learning in general terms is synonymous with meaningful discovery learning. This is learning which involves the learner sorting things out for himself by restructuring his perceptions of what is happening.'

To summarise the position adopted by those writers who devised their definitions of experiential learning from the work of Dewey would involve noting first the accent on some sort of cycle of events starting with concrete experience. It is worth noting that Kolb's and Pfeiffer and Goodstein's cycles were, in fact, anticipated by Dewey himself:

'Thinking includes all of these steps, the sense of a problem, the observation of conditions, the formation and rational elaboration of a suggested conclusion and the active experimental testing.' (Dewey, 1916)

The notion of learning from experience being a cycle involving action and reflection was a theme frequently echoed among modern writers (see for example Hampden-Turner, 1966; Kelly, 1970). Kolb's notion of transformation of experience and meaning can also be traced back to Dewey. Dewey (1938) wrote that:

'In a certain sense every experience should do something to prepare a person for later experiences of a deeper and more expansive quality. That is the very meaning of growth, continuity, reconstruction of experience.'

This, then, was the influence on experiential learning from the Dewey perspective. The accent throughout was on the primacy of personal experience and on reflection as the tool for changing knowledge and meaning.

The other main influence on the development of experiential learning was the school of psychology known as 'humanistic psychology'. Humanistic psychology developed in the 1940s, 50s and 60s as a reaction to the 'mechanism' of behavioural psychology and the determinism of psychodynamic psychology. It argued that people were free to choose their own lives and were thus 'authors' of their own existence. This philosophical perspective drew heavily on the existentialism of Sartre (1956), Heidegger (1927) and others. Humanistic psychology's main leaders, particularly in the 1960s (which offered exactly the right climate in which humanistic psychology could flourish), were Carl Rogers (1967, 1975) and Abraham Maslow (1972), who is said (Grossman, 1985) to have named humanistic psychology. Rogers is particularly well known for his client-centred counselling and for his student-centred learning methods. Many of the experiential learning methods described below developed out of the school of humanistic psychology, which, rather like Deweyan educational practices, emphasised the uniqueness of human experience and human interpretation of the world. It should be noted in passing that Rogers had been considerably influenced by Dewey as he had been taught at university by a student of Dewey's, William Kilpatrick (Kirschenbaum, 1979). In this way we begin to develop a sense of experiential learning's heritage: American (although also drawing on European philosophical traditions), with a heavy emphasis on personal experience and personal development.

THE PARTICULAR CHARACTERISTICS OF EXPERIENTIAL LEARNING

Moving on from the above discussion of experiential learning, from the theory of knowledge and from the historical perspective it is possible to draw out those characteristics that go to make up the approach to learning known as the experiential approach. These characteristics are offered as a further means of clarification and as the beginning of practical guidelines on how to use the approach. In the next chapter specific experiential learning methods will be described in detail.

In Experiential Learning there Is an Accent on Action. Both the Dewey and the humanistic approaches to experiential learning involve the learner in action. This is not to say that the learner is 'doing something' in a trivial sense but that she is engaged in an activity that should lead to learning. This is in opposition to traditional teaching/learning strategies, which require that the learner remain passive in relation to an active teacher who is the dispenser of knowledge. Freire (1972) has called this traditional approach the 'banking' approach to education: knowledge is delivered to the learner in chunks and the learner later cashes out this information during examinations. The experiential learning approach is closer to Freire's concept of 'problem posing' education. Here problems are encountered through discussion, argument and action. The learner is no longer passive but is in dialogical relationship with an equally active teacher.

There is a second, less important, sense of action too. In experiential learning the learner is often physically moving to take part in structured activities, role play, psychodrama and so on, as opposed to more traditional learning situations in which the learner sits behind a desk or table.

Learners are Encouraged to Reflect on their Experience. Most writers acknowledge that experience alone is not sufficient to ensure that learning takes place. Importance is placed on the integration of new experience with past experience through the process of reflection (Freire, 1972; Kilty, 1983; Kolb, 1984; Burnard, 1985). Reflection may be an introspective act in which the learner alone integrates new experience with old. It may also be a group process whereby sense is made of an experience through group discussion. If reflection as a group activity is to be successful, the group leader is required to act as a group facilitator and may require special skills and knowledge. These skills and types of knowledge are discussed in later chapters of this book. It is suggested that the skills associated with group facilitation are different from the skills associated with the usual processes of teaching in that the group facilitator takes a non-directive or non-authoritarian stance in relation to the learners. In a reflective group the leader as facilitator is not ascribing meanings to experience nor offering explanations, but is allowing learners to do these things for themselves.

A Phenomenological Approach Is Adopted by the Facilitator. Phenomenology may be defined as the description of objects or situations without their being ascribed values, meanings or interpretations. Phenomenology as a philosophy was developed by Husserl (1931) and underpins the philosophical writings of the existentialists (Sartre, 1956; Macquarrie, 1973).

The facilitator who uses a phenomenological approach restricts herself to the use of description as a means of summarising what a learner has said and enables that learner to invest her own learning with meaning. The 'valuing' process is left to the learner. It is the learner who ascribes meaning to what is going on in the learning environment and the facilitator's meanings are not automatically foisted on the student. Reflecting this phenomenological approach, which eschews interpretation of experience by another person, Rogers (1983) prefers to use the term 'facilitator of learning' rather than the more traditional terms 'teacher' or 'leader'. In using such a description he hoped to remove the connotation of the teacher as expert or authority in the interpretation of experience. In the literature on experiential learning the term facilitator is often used in preference to the terms 'teacher', 'lecturer', 'tutor' or 'leader'.

There Is an Accent on Subjective Human Experience. Whitehead (1933) discussed the problem of 'dead knowledge' and asserted that knowledge kept no better than fish! The experiential approach to learning stresses the evolving, dynamic nature of knowledge. Rather than evoking Peters' (1972) notion of education as initiation into particular ways of knowing, it stresses the importance of the learner understanding and creating a view of the world in that learner's *own* terms. Postman and Weingartner (1969) noted that traditional education assumes a linear model of knowledge in which there is absolute truth and a single fixed reality. Citing anthropological evidence that our language tends to limit our view of reality (Worf, 1956) and that the *means* by which subject matter is communicated fundamentally alters the *content* of that communication, Postman and Weingartner challenge the linear view of education, claiming that learners need to develop the ability to ask critical questions about any so-called 'facts' that are presented to them.

Experiential learning allows for different means of communicating concepts, accounts for 'multiple realities' and invites critical reflection. In this respect it differs considerably from the traditional model of education and training.

Human Experience Is Valued as a Source of Learning. The accent in experiential learning, through its variety of learning methods and through its name, is on experience. Learners, as has been noted, are encouraged to reflect on past experiences to plan for future events. In formulating his concept of andragogy (the theory and practice of the education of adults), Knowles (1978, 1980) stresses the value of experience in the sphere of adult learning. He maintains that as an individual matures so he accumulates an expanding reservoir of experience that causes him to become a rich resource for learning. Knowles argues that the resource should be tapped in the educational process because, as Knowles puts it, 'To an adult, his experience is *who he is*' (Knowles, 1978). Thus there is for Knowles an important ontological issue: an adult's experience is not something exterior and tacked on but is part of the person's self-concept. Experiential learning, then, is an attempt to make use of human experience as part of the learning process. It may be noted that the humanistic approach to experiential learning pays particular attention to the *emotional* aspect of the individual's experience (Heron, 1982).

Finally, while discussing the characteristics of experiential learning it may be noted that what is under consideration is:

- a set of teaching/learning methods; and
- an *attitude* towards learning.

REFERENCES

Bailey C R (1983) Experiential learning and the curriculum. *Nursing Times*, 79(29): 45–46.
Boydell T (1976) *Experiential Learning*. Manchester Monograph No. 5. Manchester: Department of Adult and Higher Education, University of Manchester.
Burnard P (1985) *Learning Human Skills: A Guide for Nurses*. London: Heinemann.
Dewey J (1916) *Democracy and Education*. New York: Free Press.
Dewey J (1938) *Experience and Education*. New York: Collier Macmillan.
FEU (1983) *Curriculum Opportunity: A Map of Experiential Learning in Entry Requirements to Higher and Further Education Award Bearing Courses*. London: Further Education Unit.
Freire P (1972) *Pedagogy of the Oppressed*. Harmondsworth: Penguin.
Grossman R (1985) Some reflections on Abraham Maslow. *Journal of Humanistic Psychology*, 25(4): 31–34.
Hampden-Turner G (1966) An existential learning theory. *Journal of Applied Behavioural Science*, 12: 4.

Heidegger M (1927) *Being and Time*. New York: Harper and Row.

Heron J (1973) *Experiential Training Techniques*. Human Potential Research Project. Guildford, Surrey: University of Surrey.

Heron J (1982) *Education of the Affect*. Human Potential Research Project. Guildford, Surrey: University of Surrey.

Husserl E (1931) *Ideas: General Introduction to Pure Phenomenology*. Translated by Boyce G. London: Allen and Unwin.

Keeton M and Associates (1976) *Experiential Learning*. San Francisco, California: Jossey Bass.

Kelly V (1970) *The Curriculum*. London: Harper and Row.

Kilty J (1983) *Experiential Learning*. Human Potential Research Project. Guildford, Surrey: University of Surrey.

Kirschenbaum H (1979) *On Becoming Carl Rogers*. New York: Dell.

Knowles M (1978) *The Adult Learner: A Neglected Species*, 2nd edn. Houston, Texas: Gulf.

Knowles M (1980) *The Modern Practice of Adult Education*, 2nd edn. Chicago: Follett.

Kolb D (1984) *Experiential Learning*. Englewood Cliffs, New Jersey: Prentice Hall.

McNulty M (1984) A framework for the future. *Nursing Mirror*, **158**: 9.

Macquarrie J (1973) *Existentialism*. Harmondsworth: Pelican.

Maslow A (1972) *Motivation and Personality*. London: Harper and Row.

Miles R (1987) Experiential learning in the curriculum. In: *The Curriculum in Nursing Education*, Allan P and Jolley M (eds.). London: Croom Helm.

Ousepensky P D (1988) *Conscience: The Search for Truth*. London: Arkana.

Peters R S (1972) Education as initiation. In: *Philosophical Analysis and Education*, Archambault R D (ed.). London: Routledge and Kegan Paul.

Pfeiffer J W and Goodstein L D (1982) *The 1982 Annual for Facilitators, Trainers and Consultants*. San Diego, California: University Associates.

Postman N and Weingartner C W (1969) *Teaching as a Subversive Activity*. Harmondsworth: Penguin.

Rogers C R (1967) *On Becoming a Person*. London: Constable.

Rogers C R (1975) *On Personal Power*. London: Constable.

Rogers C R (1983) *Freedom to Learn for the Eighties*. Columbus, Ohio: Merrill.

Sartre J-P (1956) *Being and Nothingness*. New York: Philosophical Library.

Whitehead A N (1933) *The Aims of Education*. London: Benn.

Worf B J (1983) *Language, Thought and Reality: Selected Writings*. Cambridge, Massachusetts: Technology Press of Massachusetts Institute of Technology.

CHAPTER 8

Experiential Learning Methods

There are various teaching and learning methods that may be described as experiential learning methods. Drawing on the literature on the topic (Heron, 1973; Kilty, 1983; Burnard, 1985; Kagan, 1985), the following short list of methods may be identified:

- Role play.
- Pairs activities.
- Co-counselling exercises.
- Psychodrama.
- Relaxation exercises.
- Structured group activities.
- Brainstorming.
- 'Rounds'.
- Role rehearsal.
- Encounter group activities.
- Social skills training exercises.
- Visualisation techniques.
- Meditation.

All of these methods and others are described in the literature. To give an example of the way in which such methods may be used, the variations of some of those methods and the possible pitfalls that may arise, four methods are described here: role play, brainstorming, pairs exercises and structured group activities. In recent research into the field (Burnard, 1989a), student nurses were asked to identify what they thought of as experiential learning methods used in the school of nursing; the most frequent response was 'role play'. Brainstorming represents a different but frequently used form of experiential learning in nurse education. Pairs exercises and structured group activities are particularly useful for developing interpersonal skills in nurses.

ROLE PLAY

Role play has become an accepted aspect of nurse education. Popular with tutors and sometimes less so with students, it offers a valuable and versatile means of enabling nursing students to learn aspects of the syllabus. This section considers what role play is, how it may be used and some of the problems associated with it. It also offers practical guidelines for setting up and carrying out a role play in nurse education. Well set up role play can enhance learning; poorly structured, it can put students off interactive teaching methods for life.

Role play may be usefully distinguished from skills rehearsal. Skills rehearsal involves encouraging students to practise nursing and interpersonal skills in a classroom setting. The value of such practice is clear: students may experiment and learn through doing in a safe and supportive atmosphere. It would seem realistic to practise skills before they are tried out on patients!

Role play, on the other hand, involves imagining a nursing scenario, adopting a role other than one's own and playing out a dramatisation that approximates to how things may be in a 'real' situation. Thus students may be asked to act out the roles of patients, doctors or other colleagues. This dramatic element is both the strength and the weakness of role play. Many students are put off role play because they feel that it is 'unrealistic'. Such a criticism is easily coped with. Role play *is* unrealistic! It makes no claim to being the real thing. On the other hand, the adoption of alternative behaviour can often lead us to identify strengths and skills within ourselves that we would not otherwise have recognised. In acting out a role we allow ourselves to be different. It is very easy to believe that 'this is the way I am and this is all I can do.' The truth is often that we can act and behave in various ways if we allow ourselves to.

The Uses of Role Play

For what may role play be used in nurse training? First, it can be used to explore a wide range of nursing techniques and situations, from improvising dressing techniques in difficult situations to practising coping with a distressed or aggressive relative. In this sense, it may be both a problem-solving exercise and a means of developing new skills.

Second, it can be used to enhance interpersonal competence. Basic skills such as listening and empathy building can be developed through role play, as can more advanced counselling skills (Burnard, 1989b). A mix of role play, skills rehearsal, theory input and discussion can often serve as the basis for a counselling skills workshop for both nurses in training and fieldwork teachers. Certainly, interpersonal skills can never be learned from only theoretical inputs. No-one ever learned how to communicate effectively by being lectured to. Practice of certain simple but effective skills can make the difference between the nurse who communicates and the nurse who communicates well. In this second sense role play is a form of experiential learning.

Third, role play may be used to enhance self-awareness. If we are to care for others effectively, we must come to understand ourselves better. If we are always preoccupied with our own problems, we will be unable to give our full attention to others. Neither will we be able to cope with others' emotional problems for such problems will seem too close to our own. Self-awareness training can enable us to gain insight into ourselves and help us to develop stronger and more effective coping strategies. Learning to be assertive is an example of how role play may be used to encourage self-awareness and personal skills. This use of role play is another example of experiential learning in action. The value of it, used in this way, is often enhanced if the tutor has been trained in the use of experiential learning methods prior to working with the students. The techniques and learning methods associated with experiential learning are often different from those associated with more traditional teaching methods. The Human Potential Research Project at the University of Surrey is one organisation that trains nurse tutors in a range of effective and safe experiential methods.

Finally, role play can be used to develop skills in self-presentation at interviews. As competition for jobs increases, so more and more people are becoming aware of the need for effective presentation of self during interviews. Whatever our doubts may be about the effectiveness of the interview as a selection device, the interview remains a firm favourite. We must learn, then, to cope with it effectively. Workshops can be organised in which nurses practise interview techniques in the safe and supportive atmosphere alluded to above.

Organising Role Play

Certain basic procedures are best followed if role play is to be effective. First, all participation in role play should be voluntary. No-one should be forced to take part if she does not want to. Vicarious learning often takes place through watching others, and being part of the 'audience' at a role play can do much to tell us things about ourselves. If people *are* forced to take part, they are unlikely to learn very much, except, perhaps, that they loath role play more than they thought. Very often, if people are given the option of sitting out, they will, paradoxically, feel more ready to take part. As Knowles (1975) points out, too, *all* adult learning projects should be entered into on an entirely voluntary basis. Enforced attendance at a session was probably never a very educational policy. Where role play is concerned the outcome is likely to be particularly detrimental.

Once a role play has been decided upon it needs careful structuring by the tutor, who acts as a 'director'. She must allocate roles carefully and tactfully and ensure that each player is clear about what is being asked of her. Well-structured role play enhances learning; badly run role plays are usually embarrassing.

Once the role play has been run through, it is important to evaluate it and discuss the outcomes. This can be achieved best by following this order:

- The individual players self-evaluate their performances.
- The players evaluate each other's performances.
- The 'audience' offers feedback on the players' performances.

In this way a useful balance between self- and peer evaluation is achieved. It is important that we are allowed to comment on how *we* see our work. It is also useful to find out what effect we are having on others. Often, too, we are 'saying' things to others through non-verbal communication. We can learn a lot from hearing how others interpret what we say and do.

This period of evaluation and discussion should be lengthy. Many tutors using role play for the first time tend to rush the whole procedure. This means that students do not have the chance to reflect on what has happened and to draw out the learning from it. Arguably, this reflective stage is when true learning takes place; without it, the role play just becomes 'something interesting that we did' and its educational value is diminished. A useful rule of thumb is that the evaluation and discussion should take about twice as much time as the role play itself.

After the reflective period it is helpful if the players are encouraged to re-enact the role play a second time. In this re-enactment the learning gained from the evaluation and discussion can be incorporated and reinforced. Without the second run through it is difficult to assess to what degree learning has really taken place. A second run through can also help the students to develop self-confidence in their ability to use certain positive actions and behaviours.

A variant on the standard role play is the 'perverse' role play. Here, the students are encouraged to act out their roles as *badly* as possible. The exercise can be a salutary one in that very often participants notice the similarity of what they do with 'real life'! Far from being a cause for mirth, the perverse role play can teach a great deal. It is perhaps best used within a group of students who know each other well and who are prepared to discuss the various emotions that such a role play often invokes.

There, then, are basic principles for running role play, the overriding one being to allow plenty of *time* for the activity. If such time is allowed and made use of, role play offers a valuable means of encouraging and developing the best in nursing practice.

BRAINSTORMING

The basic method of brainstorming may be described as follows. The learning group is encouraged to consider a particular topic and to call out words that they associate with it. These words are then collated onto either a black or white board or a series of flip-chart sheets. If sheets are used, they can be hung around the room to form a series of posters that serve as memory aids. During this initial process of calling out associations, the group is encouraged not to discount *any* association – often the more bizarre ones can lead to creative thinking (Koberg and Bagnall, 1981).

This process of encouraging associations can be a short one, taking, perhaps, up to 5 or 10 minutes, or it can evolve into a lengthy session of up to 40 minutes as a means of investigating a topic in depth. The noting down of associations in this way can be an end in itself. The activity can lead into a discussion or a more formal lesson. In this sense brainstorming is used as a warm-up activity to encourage initial thought about a topic.

A further elaboration of the process so far described is for the facilitator or tutor to work through the lists of words with the group, crossing out obviously inappropriate words. This is more difficult than it sounds! Often what seems inappropriate to one person is important to another!

Following this second process the facilitator can then work through the lists again with the group, in order to 'prioritise' items. Prioritising is the process of putting the items into some sort of rank order. This may mean that the items are sorted along a dimension of 'most appropriate' words to 'least appropriate' words. Out of this activity can arise the subject matter for a dis-cussion or a more formal session. The prioritised list that emerges from this activity can serve as a programme for the next session.

Another method of prioritising is to invite group members to examine the lists and to place a predetermined number of ticks against items that interest them most. Again, this method can be used to organise the next part of the programme or to determine the subject matter for the rest of the day, week, or block.

This, then, is the basic method of brainstorming, with various slight additions to make its use more extensive. The approach described above may be used in various ways. First, as we have seen, it can be used as a method of determining the content of a course. It can be used at the beginning of a workshop or on the first day of a block of training. Used in this way it ensures that the course is truly grounded in the needs and wants of the students. In this way, too, it draws upon students' prior knowledge and experience and may, therefore, be described as an experiential learning method (Hanks et al, 1977).

Second, the basic method may be used as a problem-solving device (Koberg and Bagnall, 1981; Open University, 1987). Faced with a particular clinical or practical problem in a group discussion, the tutor or facilitator may use the brainstorming approach to identify a wide range of ways of solving the problem. Again, this method calls upon the learner's prior experience and it can encourage the reinforcement of learning through practical application. It can also encourage assertive behaviour in that learners see *their* solutions written up in front of them as viable propositions.

Third, the basic method can be used as an evaluation device. At the end of a workshop or block the group is encouraged to identify their associations regarding what they have learned. These can be identified under headings such as 'knowledge' and 'skills'. Again, the process of prioritising through the use of participants' ticks can be used to identify the degree of agreement on areas of learning. The outcome of this use of brainstorming can be that new material is identified for the next learning session.

If the method is used as an evaluative process, it is important that plenty of *time* is set aside for the activity. In this way *all* aspects of learning can be identified. If the process is rushed, only the very obvious and superficial aspects of learning will surface.

Used in this way brainstorming becomes a joint evaluation/assessment process: evaluation, in that it encourages a value to be placed on what has been learned so far; assessment, in that it identifies new areas for programme planning. The process is also clearly student centred. It encourages the learners to identify what they have learned without the tutor anticipating particular areas of learning. It is worth noting, however, Paton's (1982) point that evaluation and assessment carried out in this way needs to be a very *structured* activity if it is not to degenerate into a 'free for all'. The tutor using this approach to evaluation needs to consider her level of skills in group facilitation in order to ensure that the evaluation is both systematic and effective.

Another way of using brainstorming is to consider it as a method of exploring feelings – the affective domain. Much has been written recently about the need for nurses to develop self-awareness (Burnard, 1985; Bond, 1986; Jenkins, 1987). Part of this self-awareness development comes through identifying how we *feel* about something. Thus brainstorming can become a self-awareness instrument. Two examples of its use in this way can be described.

First, it can be used as a spontaneous activity during a more formal learning session. Thus, during a session on caring for the dying person the tutor can gently encourage the group to brainstorm their feelings about the topic. Out of such a session can arise areas of personal difficulty or interest and these issues can be used as topics for further discussion. Disclosure of feeling states can also enhance self-awareness (Jourard, 1964, 1971).

Second, it can be used more directly as an 'affective activity' in its own right. Thus, the tutor sets out to explore with the group their feelings about a particular topic. For example, a group of psychiatric nursing students considering the topic of depression may be asked to identify their *own* feelings from when they have felt depressed. Again, by drawing upon the students' own past experience, used this way, brainstorming is an excellent example of an experiential learning method. This particular format is useful for exploring more 'personal' aspects of the curriculum: spirituality, sexuality, interpersonal relationships, value and belief systems and so forth.

The tutor who uses brainstorming to explore feelings in this way is recommended to have undertaken some training in facilitating the emotional release of others (Heron, 1977). The process of identifying feelings so overtly can lead to emotions being identified that had been previously suppressed or repressed. It takes tactful, patient and skilful handling by the tutor to enable students to learn from their emotional release and to gain insight from it. Handled badly, the students can be left emotionally 'raw' and may be put off future experiential learning activities. For these reasons, too, it is essential that participation of the students in these sorts of activity is always a voluntary undertaking. It seems ethically very dubious to enforce participation in learning sessions that may lead to revelation of strong feeling. Nor should any student feel that she *has* to self-disclose but should be allowed to choose her own pace and disclose only that which she feels comfortable in disclosing. The tutor who can create a safe and trusting environment can do much to help students to learn from the situation (Rogers, 1983). It should be borne in mind, too, that what is being offered to the students is an *educational* exercise and not a form of *therapy*. This is a contractual issue. Students enter a nurse training course expecting to involve themselves in educational activities and not in personal therapy.

Training in facilitating the emotional release of others is increasingly being offered by colleges and extramural departments of universities, and tutors may wish to consider such training as part of their refresher courses. Others may wish to consider longer-term training in psychodynamic training, such as is offered by the Tavistock Institute in London.

Finally, two variants of the basic method of brainstorming may be considered. One is the use of brainstorming as a small group activity (Newble and Cannon, 1987). Students are invited to form into small groups of three to five members. In each group a facilitator or chairperson is elected and that person serves as the one who writes down the associations on flip-chart sheets. After a period of about 15 minutes the small groups re-form and a plenary session is held. In this session each group pins up its sheets and all other participants are invited to view the displayed sheets. Out of this viewing period evolves a discussion of a more general sort. The advantage of this approach to brainstorming is that it allows almost everyone to take part. Students who are more reticent in a large group may feel more comfortable working in a small one.

The second variant on the basic approach is that of 'individual' brainstorming. Here, students are encouraged to sit quietly on their own and write down all the associations that they make on a particular topic. When a given period of time has passed (usually between 5 and 10 minutes) these students may be invited to form a plenary session. In this session two things may be done. One is to discuss the *process* of the activity, i.e. what it *felt like* to carry out the activity. Second is to invite students to share what they have written down. This, again, must be a voluntary activity. Some of the jottings may be of a personal nature and group members may or may not wish to share them with the whole group.

Used in this way the process of brainstorming becomes akin to the process of free-association – the basic activity of psychoanalysis (Hall, 1954; Bullock and Stallybrass, 1977). Perhaps because of this, strong feelings may, again, be identified. Again, it is recommended that tutors using this method develop skills in handling emotions. It should, of course, be emphasised that this form of brainstorming is only *similar* to one aspect of psychoanalysis. Clearly it is nothing to do with psychoanalysis itself in that psychoanalysis is a structured and lengthy therapeutic process that involves interpretation, by a trained analyst, of the associations made by the client. It is not suggested that brainstorming should evolve into a form of do-it-yourself psychoanalysis.

Certain principles emerge from all the different sorts of brainstorming activity described here and out of the literature cited above. They may be enumerated as follows:

1. Keep it simple but keep it structured. Instructions need to be given clearly and be easily understood. The structure of the activity serves to keep that activity focused.
2. Keep to time. If the activity overruns, it may appear loose and unstructured. If it underruns, it may appear rushed.
3. Ensure that all associations are written down exactly as they are offered by the students. It is important that the tutor does not offer an 'interpretation' of students' offerings.
4. Allow everyone to have their say. It is important that domination by one student is kept to a minimum and that all feel free to talk.

PAIRS EXERCISES

Pairs exercises are particularly useful for learning and practising interpersonal skills such as counselling skills. The usual format for the pairs exercise is that each person nominates themselves A or B. Then A practises the particular skill (for example, using open-ended questions) in the supportive presence of B. After a period in these roles the two people swap round and B practises the skill in the supportive presence of A. It is important that the exercise is *not* seen as a form of conversation but as a highly structured learning exercise. After each of the individuals has had a turn in the driving seat the pair may spend time freely evaluating and appraising the exercise. Alternatively, the pair may rejoin a larger group to discuss the exercise with other people.

An alternative use of the pairs format is for the pair in question to take a theme and for one person to discuss that theme while the other person listens. After a prescribed time the pair switch roles and the listener becomes the talker and vice versa. After an equal amount of time in this second phase of the activity the pair may link up with another pair and discuss the issue in a foursome. Alternatively, they may be invited back into a larger group to discuss the issues among their colleagues.

STRUCTURED GROUP ACTIVITIES

Structured group exercises allow for the experiential learning cycle to be worked through by a learning group. There are a number of publications that describe a variety of group activities for enhancing interpersonal, social and counselling skills (Murgatroyd, 1986; Burnard, 1989b). The idea of these activities is that the group undertakes an experience after which the members discuss their thoughts and feelings about the experience and apply the new learning to the real or clinical situation. The advantages of this approach include the sharing of a common experience, the generation of a wide range of possible solutions to practical problems and the realisation of both the personal and the common nature of group experience. Much can be learnt, experientially, about how to run and to be members of groups by taking part in structured group activities. Many of the best structured group activities are those that the facilitator or the group devise themselves.

There are some important guidelines that may help in the smooth running of structured group activities that may be identified as follows:

- Full and clear instructions must be given to the group and questions asked by the facilitator to establish that everyone in the group is clear about what to do.
- Participation should always be voluntary and participants should be given the chance to sit out as observers.
- Plenty of time must be set aside *after* the exercise in order to 'process' or discuss the activity. Rushed processing of activities is a sure sign of an inexperienced facilitator.
- The facilitator should be just that and not rush to offer her own explanations or interpretations of what has just happened in the group.
- A debriefing period should follow the exercise to allow time for the participants to re-enter their normal, everyday roles.
- The facilitator should encourage the group members to link any new learning with 'real life' and with their jobs away from the group. Group members should also be encouraged to practise any new skills learned as soon as possible.

These are some basic experiential learning methods and a number of variants. All of them have been used by one of the present writers in a variety of contexts, including psychiatric nurse train-

ing, undergraduate and postgraduate nursing degree programmes, post-basic and continuing education activities and a
wide range of interpersonal skills and counselling workshops.
Clearly, many other applications exist beyond those described here
and many such applications will arise out of the tutor's experience.
Many of the best experiential learning activities are those that
are invented during a paticular programme. Such invention adds
freshness and vitality to a learning encounter and must, by its
very nature, be student-centred – centred on *this* group at *this*
time.

REFERENCES

Bond M (1986) *Stress and Self-Awareness: A Guide for Nurses*. London:
Heinemann.
Bullock A and Stallybrass O (1977) *The Fontana Dictionary of Modern
Thought*. London: Fontana/Collins.
Burnard P (1985) *Learning Human Skills: A Guide for Nurses*. London:
Heinemann.
Burnard P (1989a) Psychiatric nursing students' perception of experiential
learning. *Nursing Times*, 85(1): 52.
Burnard P (1989b) *Counselling Skills for Health Professionals*. London: Chap-
man and Hall.
Hall C (1955) *A Primer of Freudian Psychology*. New York: New American
Library.
Hanks L, Belliston L and Edwards D (1977) *Design Yourself*. Los Altos,
California: Kaufmann.
Heron J (1973) *Experiential Training Techniques*. Human Potential Research
Project. Guildford, Surrey: University of Surrey.
Heron J (1977) *Catharsis in Human Development*. Human Potential Research
Project. Guildford, Surrey: University of Surrey.
Jenkins E (1987) *Facilitating Self Awareness: A Learning Package Combining
Group Work with Computer Assisted Learning*. Wigan: Open Software
Library.
Jourard S (1964) *The Transparent Self*. New Jersey: Van Nostrand.
Jourard S (1971) *Self-disclosure: An Experiential Analysis of the Transparent
Self*. New York: Wiley.
Kagan C (ed.) (1985) *Interpersonal Skills in Nursing: Research and Applications*.
London: Croom Helm.
Kilty J (1983) *Experiential Learning*. Human Potential Research Project.
Guildford, Surrey: University of Surrey.
Knowles M (1975) *Self-Directed Learning*. New York: Cambridge.
Knowles M (1980) *The Modern Practice of Adult Education*, 2nd edn. Chicago:
Follett.
Koberg D and Bagnall J (1981) *The Revised All New Universal Traveler: A*

Soft-systems Guide to Creativity, Problem-solving and the Process of Reaching Goals. Los Altos, California: Kaufmann.

Murgatroyd S (1986) *Counselling and Helping*. London: Methuen.

Newble D and Cannon R (1987) *A Handbook for Medical Teachers*, 2nd edn. Lancaster: MTP Press.

Open University, Coping With Crisis Research Group (1987) *Running Workshops: A Guide for Trainers in the Helping Professions*. London: Croom Helm.

Paton M Q (1982) *Practical Evaluation*. Beverly Hills, California: Sage.

Rogers C R (1983) *Freedom to Learn for the Eighties*. Columbus, Ohio: Merrill.

CHAPTER 9

The Mentor System in Nurse Education

In learning and developing nursing skills we all need help at times. Sometimes it is useful if the help regularly comes from the same person and we can develop a lasting relationship with that helper. It is here that we find the basis of the notion of mentoring. The idea of having a mentor during health-care training received considerable attention in the American press (Attwood, 1979; May et al, 1982), and two writers go as far as to say that 'everyone who makes it has a mentor' (Collins and Scott, 1979). Burton (1975) notes that many of the famous American playwrights and poets revealed that they had mentors at some stage in their careers. In this country the notion has been less written about but is gaining momentum in the health-care professions as a format for developing interpersonal skills in health professionals. In Torbay Health Authority (Morris et al, 1988), for example, the mentor relationship has been used with considerable success in working out a new style of psychiatric nurse education.

What, then, are mentors, why do we need them and how do we train them? A mentor is usually someone older than the student who has considerable experience of the job for which the student is being prepared. The idea of having a mentor usually also contains the notion of continuity and of the student staying with the mentor for some time. This is in contrast to more traditional approaches to health professionals' education, where continuity with teaching staff is necessarily interrupted by field experience and where students work with a qualified person for only a short period of time. With the mentor system trainees negotiate who their mentor will be and then stay 'allocated' to that person for the length of their training. Necessarily, then, a closer relationship is likely to develop between the mentor and student than has traditionally been the case.

Darling (1984) found in her research that there were three 'absolute requirements for a significant mentoring relationship'. These were attraction, action and affect. In the first instance, attraction, it is deemed vital that both people respect and like each other. Arguably, as the relationship develops a *transference* relationship will evolve (Burton, 1977). The term 'transference' is usually reserved as a descriptor for the nature of the relationship that develops between a psychotherapist and her client. It signifies that the client comes to see the therapist as having personal characteristics (usually positive ones) that are reminiscent of one of the client's parents. All this normally takes place at a pre- or unconscious level so the client does not readily see that this is happening. The net result is usually that the client 'idealises' the therapist and becomes very dependent on her. One of the aims of therapy is often to help the client to try to resolve this transference relationship and thus live a less dependent and more interdependent life (Burnard, 1989). It seems likely that the relationship between student and mentor is also likely to invoke transference, particularly as the mentor is already cast in the role of 'expert' by the very nature of being a mentor at all. All this suggests that mentors should be chosen very carefully. Who should do this 'choosing' remains a question for debate.

It is possible, too, that the 'attraction' could include emotional and sexual attraction. The ethical position here is clear – at least in theory. The relationship between mentor and student should remain a 'Platonic' one, given the tacit contract that exists between teachers, clinical staff and students. Life is rarely as simple as that, however, and the issue of how to cope with more involved relationships clearly needs addressing.

In terms of the 'action' role of the mentor, the student is likely to want to use the mentor as a role model. Again, by definition, the mentor is seen as an expert: someone who has achieved the various skills that are deemed necessary for effective practice and who is able to use and pass on those skills. In a sense this aspect of mentoring may be equivalent to the 'sitting with Nellie' approach to training office staff in some organisations. 'Sitting with Nellie' refers to the idea of learning skills by sitting with and watching the person who has them. Clearly, though, it is to be hoped that this will not be the only way that skills are passed on. Traditionally, there has been an element of this approach in training approaches for students. Just being with a qualified person was sometimes seen as enough to encourage and enable students to develop various skills. Whether or not this *was* ever the case is another debatable point. A certain skill in coaching seems to be a requirement of the skilled mentor. The ability to break down skills into component parts and teach them, and the ability to demonstrate their use with the appropriate, accompanying affect seems to be another skill to aim for. Mentoring, it would seem, is not for the faint hearted.

From the 'affective' point of view, the mentor needs to act in a supportive role. She should be able to encourage the student, enhance her self-confidence and teach her to be constructively critical of what she sees and does. Again, this aspect of the role is likely to re-open the debate about the likelihood of a transference relationship occurring. If transference does occur, it is important that the mentor be able to cope with it. She will also need to know how to close the relationship and be skilled in 'saying goodbye'. This is unlikely to be easy because of the possible counter-transference, i.e. the mentor's complicated network of feelings for the student, that may occur. At best, however, the relationship may come to mirror the best aspects of the truly therapeutic relationship that the student will develop with her patients. Hopefully, then, the mentor will be able to initiate and sustain the sort of exemplary relationship that will stand as a role model for future relationships. Again, a lot is being asked of the person who acts as mentor.

If such a relationship *does* develop and is sustained, it is likely to be very valuable for the student and, no doubt, for the mentor. If the heart of nursing is concerned with relationships, a close relationship between one who 'knows' and one who is learning may be useful to both and, subsequently, to the patients.

On the other hand, there are numerous problems. Because of the nature of the partnership the student starts in a 'one-down' relationship with the mentor. The mentor is necessarily in a dominant position in the relationship. It is not and cannot be a relationship of equals. Now much of the recent writing on adult education has suggested that adult education should concern itself with negotiation, with shared learning and with meeting students' own perceived needs (Brookfield, 1987). Adults, so this argument goes, need to *use* what they learn as they learn it; they need to be treated as equals in a partnership that leads along a road of inquiry; and they need to have their self-concept protected as they go. Whether or not such demands for equality and negotiation can exist within the constraints of the mentor–student relationship is not clear. It seems more likely that the mentor will be identified as a benign (or perhaps, not so benign) father or mother substitute. Some may find such a portrayal overdramatic but, as we have noted, the perfectly respectable notion of transference depends upon the 'unconscious designation' of the other person as a surrogate parent.

There is also the problem of the mentor's own development. There is nothing worse than the 'guru' who feels that she has gained enlightenment and that all she needs to do is sit back and pass on pearls of wisdom to others. I write 'she': unfortunately, such guru figures are nearly always male. All of us need to continue our development and education. None of us has 'arrived'; none of us is skilled to the point where we cannot learn other skills. The mentor must be a convert to, if anything, lifelong education (Gross, 1977).

Lifelong education is a concept that fits in well with the notion of experiential learning. With lifelong learning the assumption is that education does not and should not end with 'formal' education. Unfortunately, the preparation of many health-care professionals is such that a 'front-end' model of education and training is offered. That is to say that there is a lengthy preparation period (often of between 2 and 6 years), followed by very little further education apart from the occasional study day. The responsibility for further and continuing education thus becomes the responsibility of the individual practitioner. This is particularly pertinent to the mentor who will be responsible for helping the newcomer to the profession. Lifelong learning commends an approach entailing personal responsibility for learning. Gross (1977) in his introductory text *The Lifelong Learner* sums up this approach as follows:

> 'This idea of self-development is the link between your life and learning. A free learner seizes the exhilarating responsibility for the growth of his or her own mind. This starts when you realise that you must decide what you will make of yourself.'

Lifelong learning is concerned with growth and development. There are echoes here of Whitehead's (1933) remark, quoted above: 'knowledge keeps no better than fish!' The lifelong learner is one who does not hoard 'dead knowledge' but appreciates the changing nature of it. What serves us well as knowledge and skill today will, to quite an extent, be out of date tomorrow. No health professional can afford to allow her knowledge and skill base to become out of date. Interestingly, the task of being a mentor can help in the process of keeping up to date as the mentor also learns from the person for whom she is mentor. This raises an interesting paradox. While the mentor takes responsibility for overseeing the learner, she must also be constantly consulting that learner about how she will determine the next part of her learning. The mentor, in other words, should always be trying to do herself out of a job.

All these things, and no doubt plenty more, need consideration before the partnership of mentoring begins. Alternatively, they could be faced as they occur, which may be the more painful way.

How can mentors be trained? *Should* they be trained? There is a tendency, in some quarters, to be disparaging about training in the interpersonal domain. Some prefer to think of health professionals as having 'natural' ability in their field. It would seem reasonable, however, to try to identify some of the aspects of the role that would lend themselves to training.

First, the mentor will need skills in identifying learning objectives with the student. This involves skilful negotiation of the student's objectives. Such negotiations takes two factors into account: what the student identifies as a need and what the mentor identifies as a need. Together the two people must work out a reasonable and workable programme.

Second, mentors will need to be interpersonally competent. This means that they will be able to initiate and maintain a student-centred relationship that takes full account of the possibility of transference occurring. They will be skilled as counsellors and be prepared to set aside a regular time to talk to the student. This aspect of the role may be described as the 'befriending' aspect.

Third, mentors will need coaching skills. They will require the ability, described above, to encourage learning. This is, of course, different from the skills required of a teacher, for mentors will not be teachers in the traditional sense of the term. Students will, however, by various means, learn a great deal from them.

Finally in this tentative list of requirements, the mentor will need skills in enabling the student to self-evaluate – both the student's skills and the nature of the mentor–student relationship. Thus, the mentor will be encouraging the development of self-awareness in the student. Such awareness is likely to help the student in her subsequent relationships with patients or clients. All in all, the relationship needs to be an unselfish one on the part of the mentor.

These, then, are some of the issues involved in the concept of mentoring. What is not clear at the moment is the degree to which mentoring will become commonly adopted within the structure of nursing education. Two obvious problems arise when discussing the notion of mentoring. First, it is possible to question the notion that someone can be *designated* a mentor. While we can all recall people that have made a significant difference to our development at various points throughout our careers, these people have usually 'emerged'. No-one ever said to us that they would be a significant influence. Indeed, it is possible to look back and be surprised at the people who served us as mentors and to realise that we may not necessarily have chosen them as mentors at the time. Thus, the question needs to be raised about the wisdom of prescribing mentors for other people.

The second problem arises out of whether or not mentoring is compatible with student-centred learning. Throughout this book and throughout much of the current literature on nurse education is the recurrent theme of encouraging learners to become autonomous, to learn to become independent of their tutors and to develop their critical ability. Such a notion is a reasonable one. If nurses are to develop beyond their basic training and education (whatever form that may take), they need to develop the skills of independent learning that lead to independent thinking. Now, it may be argued that the notion of mentoring asks that learners become *dependent* upon their mentors. The idea of the mentor, as we have noted, involves a number of criteria, which Collins (1983) identifies as follows:

'The mentor is:

- an authority in the field,
- an influential figure,
- interested in growth and development,
- committed to the relationship,
- organisationally higher placed than the mentee.'

There may be a conflict of aims and interests in, on the one hand, arguing that nurse learners should gain independence fairly rapidly and, on the other hand, contriving a relationship with a more senior person in which the learner necessarily plays out the role of apprentice. It will be interesting to note the degree to which the idea of mentoring becomes part of the larger debate about nurse education in the final decades of nurse education in this century.

REFERENCES

Attwood A H (1979) The mentor in clinical practice. *Nursing Outlook*, **27**: 714–717.
Brookfield S (1987) *Developing Critical Thinkers: Challenging Adults to Explore Alternative Ways of Thinking and Acting*. Milton Keynes: Open University Press.
Burnard P (1989) *Counselling Skills for Health Professionals*. London: Chapman and Hall.
Burton A (1975) The mentoring dynamic in the therapeutic transformation. *The American Journal of Psychoanalysis*, **37**: 115–122.
Collins R L (1983) *Professional Women and their Mentors*. Englewood Cliffs, New Jersey: Prentice Hall.
Collins G C and Scott P (1979) Everyone who makes it has a mentor. *Harvard Business Review*, **56**: 89–101.
Darling L A W (1984) What do nurses want in a mentor? *The Journal of Nursing Administration*, **14**(10): 42–44.
Gross R (1977) *The Lifelong Learner*. New York: Simon and Schuster.
May K M et al (1982) Mentorship for scholarliness: opportunities and dilemmas. *Nursing Outlook*, **30**: 22–28.
Morris N, John G and Keen T (1988) Learning the ropes. *Nursing Times*, **84**(16): 24–27.
Whitehead A N (1933) *The Aims of Education*. London: Benn.

CHAPTER 10

Evaluating Learning in Nurse Education

Traditional methods of evaluation in nurse education have been discussed at length elsewhere (see for example Allan and Jolley, 1982). Many evaluation methods describe evaluation as something only to be carried out by nurse educators. In other words, the students are the passive recipients of education and all that remains is for their teachers to test out whether or not the educational experience has worked. On the other hand, as we have noted, there is a growing trend towards student-centred learning and towards learners taking responsibility for their own learning. If this is the case, it would seem logically wrong to exclude them from some decision-making in the evaluation process. We cannot argue for freedom and responsibility in learning and for learner autonomy and at the same time remove that freedom, responsibility and autonomy from the evaluation process. Here, we consider self- and peer assessment as appropriate methods of evaluating the sorts of educational programme discussed in this book. It is not suggested that self- and peer assessment should be the *only* means of evaluating learning but that they may be used effectively *alongside* other methods. Currently, schools of nursing have the responsibility for setting their own final examinations, and this may create a tension between the student-centred approach on the one hand and the need to set an 'objective' examination on the other.

There is a growing literature on the use of self- and peer assessment and evaluation (Kilty, 1977; Heron, 1982; Burnard, 1987). With the increase in interest in experiential learning is coming the realisation that those taking part in adult learning groups need to be able to develop their own criteria for checking and evaluating their own learning (Knowles, 1975, 1978, 1980). In this section the use of one such student-centred approach is discussed: the journal as a method of self-assessment and evaluation.

Self-evaluation can be a means of identifying personal progress. It can enable the nurse to clarify what she has learned and how past learning can be incorporated with present. In this sense, it is a process of synthesis.

It can also enable the learner to identify gaps in her learning and development. This can help in the setting of new learning goals and in making economical use of time and resources. If the learner never self-evaluates, she tends to 'carry on as usual', not noting whether she has progressed or regressed. There is also a tendency for the learner to continue to cover the same ground: perhaps we all prefer to stick to what we know. Self-evaluation, then, can enable the learner to stop and take stock in order to prepare herself for further learning.

The process of self-evaluation can also be an integral part of self-awareness development. As we shall see, one aspect of self-evaluation involves inviting feedback from others. That feedback can encourage the learner to develop a balanced self-image. We need others to tell us who we are. In this sense, self-awareness becomes a two-way process: it invokes a reflective, inward looking aspect, yet also calls for the learner to take note of other people's views. Such a balanced view satisfies both the self-disclosure and feed-back-from-others requirements that Luft (1969) argues are essential for self-awareness.

Self- and peer evaluation are also means of developing autonomy in learning (Boud, 1981). If a student becomes totally dependent upon other people's evaluation of her progress, she will tend to deny the importance of her own evaluation. When evaluation by others is the only sort allowed, students begin to believe that educational 'experts' are the only ones who are able to evaluate effectively. Then tests, examinations, certificates and diplomas become the only valid means of appreciating that learning has taken place.

Alternatively, the student who can effectively self-evaluate can become an independent learner. She can begin the process of 'valuing herself', of appreciating that a person's own evaluation of her performance is, in the end, one of the most important aspects of the educational process.

It is acknowledged that the two concepts of assessment and evaluation are inextricably linked. To assess is to identify a particular state at a particular time, usually with a view to taking action to change or modify that state. To evaluate is to place a value on a course of action, to identify the success or otherwise of something that has happened. Thus, assessment is often seen as something that needs to occur at the outset of an educational encounter and evaluation as something that occurs at the end. In fact, evaluation necessarily leads on to reassessment and thus to another educational encounter.

There are limits to self-evaluation. Summative evaluation (Scriven, 1967) carried out by an objective person or body is an important aspect of professional education. However, once entry into the profession has been achieved or once a degree or diploma has been obtained, self-monitoring through self-evaluation becomes the more autonomous and mature means of further development. We cannot expect to rely on other people's evaluation of our ability for evermore, so it would seem important to get used to the self- and peer evaluation approach as early as possible. In a sense, of course, we are self-evaluating all the time: I am monitoring and checking what I am writing, as I write it; you are checking what you are reading against your own beliefs and values as you read.

METHODS OF SELF-EVALUATION

Various methods of self-evaluation are identified in the educational literature (Rowntree, 1977; Sullivan, 1977; Clift and Imrie, 1981). Questionnaires and ranking and rating scales may be used as methods of self-evaluation (Fink and Kosecoff, 1978; Narayanasamy, 1985; Reynolds and Cormack, 1985). In this chapter, as illustrations of the self and peer approach to nurse education, we consider various practical methods: the use of the journal and a variety of individual and group procedures for self- and peer evaluation.

The Journal

A modified version of the journal has been used at the School of Nursing Studies, University of Wales College of Medicine, as part of a continuous assessment procedure during the students' psychiatric nursing secondment of the Bachelor of Nursing course. It has met with varying amounts of success. After an initial period of the students' feeling that they would not be able to complete the journal, a number found it particularly useful and planned to continue to use it throughout other parts of their course. Others continued to find it difficult to use and one never completed it.

The instructions for completion of the journal are simple. Participants are required to make weekly entries in a suitable book under the following headings:

- Problems encountered and resolution of those problems.
- Application of new skills and difficulties with them.
- New skills required to be learned.
- Personal growth issues/self-awareness development.
- Other comments.

These headings can be varied according to the needs and wants of a particular group using the journal approach. No guidelines need to be given regarding the amount that is written under each heading. To prescribe a particular number of words would be over-structuring, although it may be possible to *negotiate* maxima and minima with the group.

Participants are encouraged to make regular entries and this regularity tends to make the process of keeping the diary easier. Participants who try to 'catch up' and complete the whole thing in one last go tend to have difficulty in remembering what has happened and generally the process is less valuable.

There are several methods of using the diary as an assessment/evaluation tool. The first is to use it in an on-going group as a continuous focus of discussion between the facilitator and the group. In this way the participants' experience is constantly being monitored and they are able to discuss their progress or lack of it as they continue with day-to-day field work.

The second method is to use it as a means of summative evaluation at the end of a period of field work (Scriven, 1967). In this case, the following procedure may be used:

- Both facilitator and student sit down and individually 'brainstorm' criteria for assessing the journal. Examples of items brainstormed may be:

  – quality of writing;

  – clarity of expression;
  – ability to problem-solve;
  – level of self-disclosure.

- After this brainstorming session, both facilitator and participant identify three criteria that they wish to use as criteria
  for assessing the journal.
- Each then uses those criteria to write notes on their assessment of the journal, and they then compare those notes.

Out of this activity comes a shared view of the journal, which
incorporates elements of both self- and facilitator evaluation. The
discussion that follows can be useful to both participants and
facilitator as a means of offering further feedback on performance.
This method can also be used to focus on another important
communication skill: the written word. This is a particularly fruit-
ful area if the participant is, in this case, a student or trainee in
the health-care field. At this stage, too, a mark for the diary can be
negotiated if the journal is to form part of a continuous assessment
procedure.

A third method of using the journal is as part of a weekly discussion. This can serve as a means of focusing on shared problems
and also as a method of disseminating new information and learning. The journal can also form the basis of a seminar group, with
each member in turn taking the lead to run the group.

Probably the most democratic method of deciding how to use the
journal is to negotiate that use with the group. This should be
done prior to the journal being undertaken so that all participants
are clear as to who will and who will not have access to it. Journal
writing calls for a considerable degree of self-disclosure and it is
important in adult learning groups that the participants' dignity
is maintained (Jarvis, 1983).

The journal as part of a total assessment and evaluation system
in nurse training can be a valuable and very personal means of
participants' maintaining a constant check on their own learning
and development. The approach can be modified in a variety of
ways to reflect different emphases. For instance, the bias can be
towards practical skills development, or towards self-awareness.
Alternatively, participants can be encouraged to develop their own
headings for the journal in order to reflect their own needs and
wants.

It is interesting to consider the various levels of assessment and evaluation that take place when this method is used. First, the participants have to reflect on their experience before they write. Second, they have to convert their thoughts into words and write an entry in the journal. Third, another level of assessment occurs when the journal is discussed between other group members or in a tutorial. In this way participants are completing part of the experiential learning cycle discussed in Chapter 7. They are also fulfilling the conditions of self-disclosure and feedback from others that Luft (1969) considers necessary for the development of self-awareness. Thus, the method offers a valuable educational tool on a number of levels.

There are other methods of self- and peer evaluation and some of these will be described briefly.

Self-evaluation
Perhaps the simplest form of self-evaluation is for the learner to sit down and write out a few pages that illustrate her acknowledgement of her progress to date. This 'freehand' sketch may then be used as the basis of a discussion with another learner or with a tutor. This form of self-evaluation has the advantage of allowing the learner to decide what she feels to be important in terms of evaluation and allows her to choose the areas that she evaluates. It has the disadvantage that it is not systematic and is a purely subjective description of one person's view of her learning.

Self- and Peer Evaluation – 1
A simple method of introducing self- and peer evaluation is to use the programme as a basis of evaluation. Here, the students sit down with a copy of the day or week's programme and, individually, write out comments on their own learning performance in each of the sessions. These appraisals are then discussed in the group and colleagues are invited to give individuals feedback on their performance. Thus, this second aspect of the self- and peer evaluation procedure will start with one learner reading out her comments about her learning that week. Then she will invite the group to offer comments about her performance during that week, thus satisfying the 'peer' aspect of the evaluation. This type of self- and peer evaluation has the advantage of being more systematic than the previous evaluation device. It allows for peer feedback as well as for individual commentary. It has the disadvantage of taking time to undertake thoroughly. Arguably, though, the procedure allows the locus of control in evaluation to move away

from the nurse educator towards the individual learner and her peers.

Self- and Peer Evaluation – 2
More formal self- and peer evaluation is an activity that can easily be carried out in a small learning group. The stages of the process are identified in Figure 10.1.

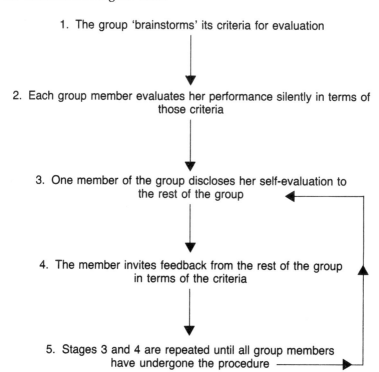

1. The group 'brainstorms' its criteria for evaluation

2. Each group member evaluates her performance silently in terms of those criteria

3. One member of the group discloses her self-evaluation to the rest of the group

4. The member invites feedback from the rest of the group in terms of the criteria

5. Stages 3 and 4 are repeated until all group members have undergone the procedure

Figure 10.1 Stages in self- and peer evaluation

First, the group of learners meets and brainstorms its criteria for self- and peer evaluation. Examples of such criteria are performance in the group, knowledge level, expression of opinions, feelings or values and leadership qualities. The nature of the criteria chosen will depend on context: the small seminar group will probably generate different criteria from the larger learning group.

Once the criteria for evaluation have been decided upon by consensus, the group splits up so that individual members can silently evaluate their own performance in terms of the criteria. It is helpful if this evaluation is written down so that individual learners have something concrete to refer to in the later discussion. This stage of the process may take between 10 minutes and half an hour depending on the number of criteria decided upon.

The group then re-forms and one of the learners starts the procedure by disclosing her own evaluation according to the criteria. This should be complete and uninterrupted by other members of the group. If time is a major consideration, it may be suggested that each person takes no more than 10 minutes over this stage of the evaluation process. Otherwise, it is far more effective if no time limit is set.

The first person then invites feedback from the group on her performance in terms of the criteria. All negative feedback should be given first, followed by positive feedback. In this way, the negative issues are dealt with initially and the individual closes this aspect of the evaluation process feeling positive.

There is a definite skill in giving feedback to others. It should be offered 'cleanly' – negative feedback should not degenerate into a personal attack on the other person: it should aim, instead, at offering useful and constructive observations of that person's behaviour. Nor should positive feedback be unnecessarily qualified. It is all too easy to offer someone a positive observation followed by an unnerving and negative 'but. . .'!

Again, if time is limited, the group feedback for one person may be completed in 5 or 10 minutes. There is considerable value, however, in taking time over this aspect of the evaluation process and, wherever possible, such time constraints should not be used.

When one person has completed the cycle of self-evaluation and has received feedback from the group, another person works through the cycle until all have undergone the process. It is important that everyone takes part, including the lecturer or tutor, although it is wise to make the 'peer' aspect optional. Not everyone wants or needs comments on their performance from other people, although experience suggests that many people *do* benefit from it.

The facilitator's role is to manage the sequence of events. In the brainstorming of criteria the facilitator keeps the group to the task in hand and prevents one member from lionising it. It is not part of the facilitator's job to have the last word nor to summarise the comments offered by the group to a particular member. In this democratic process it is important that the facilitator is not a chair-person but is only there to see that the group is aware of the timing and stages of the process. Indeed, once the group has become used to the procedure the facilitator's role becomes redun-dant and the group itself manages the whole process, further affirming the underlying egalitarian principle.

These, then, are a number of approaches to the process of self- and peer evaluation. As we have noted, they need not be used exclusively but can be combined with more traditional 'objective' approaches to educational evaluation in order to create an imagin-ative mix of the objective and subjective.

REFERENCES

Allan P and Jolley M (1982) *Nursing, Midwifery and Health Visiting since 1900.* London: Faber and Faber.
Boud D (ed.) (1981) *Developing Student Autonomy in Learning.* London: Kogan Page.
Burnard P (1987) Self and peer assessment. *Senior Nurse,* **6**(5): 16–17.
Clift J C and Imrie B W (1981) *Assessing Students: Appraising Teaching.* London: Croom Helm.
Fink A and Kosecoff J (1978) *An Evaluation Primer.* London: Sage.
Heron J (1982) *Assessment.* Human Potential Research Project. Guildford, Surrey: University of Surrey.
Jarvis P (1983) *The Theory and Practice of Adult and Continuing Education.* London: Croom Helm.
Kilty J (1977) *Self and Peer Assessment.* Human Potential Research Project. Guildford, Surrey: University of Surrey.
Knowles M (1975) *Self-Directed Learning.* New York: Cambridge.
Knowles M (1978) *The Adult Learner: A Neglected Species,* 2nd edn. Texas: Gulf.
Knowles M (1980) *The Modern Practice of Adult Education.* Chicago: Follett.
Luft J (1969) *Of Human Interaction: The Johari Model of Interaction.* Palo Alto, California: Mayfield.
Narayanasamy S A (1985) Evaluation of a training curriculum for nursing assistants. *Nurse Education Today,* **5**(3): 124–129.
Reynolds W and Cormack D F S (1985) Clinical teaching of group dynam-ics: an evaluation of a trial clinical teaching programme. *Nurse Education Today,* **5**(3): 101–108.
Rowntree D (1977) *Assessing Students: How Shall We Know Them?* London: Harper and Row.

Scriven M (1967) The methodology of evaluation. In: *Perspectives of Curriculum Evaluation*, Tyler R W (ed.). Chicago: Rand McNally.

Sullivan A M (1977) A framework for the evaluation of teaching: self assessment and formal evaluation. In: *If Teaching Is Important: The Evaluation of Instruction in Higher Education*, Knapper C K, Geis G L, Pascal C E and Shore B H (eds.). Canadian Association of University Teachers, Toronto: Clark, Irwin and Co.

PART III

Towards the Future: Trends and Developments

CHAPTER 11

Project 2000

In 1986 the UKCC issued a document entitled *Project 2000: A New Preparation for Practice*. This was the result of a working group set up by the UKCC, which contained representatives of the various disciplines within nursing, representatives of further and higher education and members from the UKCC and the four National Boards. During the deliberations of this group, members consulted widely with the profession by issuing papers on specific topics and by conducting 'road shows'. Feedback from both of these activities was incorporated into a document that went out for final consultation to the profession. The final recommendations, when issued, were seen to be a joint exercise between the five Statutory Bodies – the UKCC and the four National Boards – and as such were presented to representatives of Government from the four countries of the UK.

As part of the work required by the working group a firm of management consultants (Price Waterhouse) was commissioned to collect information on manpower requirements, recruitment, wastage, etc. This the firm did by gathering facts and figures, constructing computer models and using a health authority in each of the four countries for case history purposes.

During this investigation a worrying demographic feature was highlighted, the fact that the number of 18-year-olds is declining to a low point that will be reached in 1995, when, based on the current figures, there will be a potential shortfall of approximately 3000 recruits to the profession, with an accumulated shortfall by the year 2000 of 10 000 nurse practitioners. This 'demographic time-bomb' emphasised the urgent need to reduce wastage and to make more effective use of nurses entering the profession.

Another feature highlighted at this time was the dissatisfaction of the enrolled nurse, who was often used as a substitute for the registered nurse despite the fact that enrolled nurse training was inadequate as preparation for that position, had no real possibility of career progression and in the words commonly used at the time was 'abused and misused'.

Obviously, to understand fully the proposals contained in the Project 2000 document the whole paper needs to be read; however, for the purpose of discussion they can be summarised under the headings below.

EDUCATION

In order to produce an educated individual able to react to rapidly changing health-care needs – a 'knowledgeable doer' – and to reduce duplication in training programmes as well as wastage from nurse training, the following were proposed.

One Level of Qualified (Registered) Nurse

In order to achieve this, state enrolled nurse training was to be discontinued and those enrolled nurses who so wished and were able to do so were to be offered 'conversion' courses to enable them to reach registration status. There would also be a change in the emphasis of nursing education.

In future, education was to be rooted in health not disease, with an increased emphasis on health education and preventative care. It was also recommended that the registered nurse be prepared to function equally well outside as inside institutions.

Changes in the Pattern of Nursing Education

The proposal was for a 'common foundation programme' lasting 2 years which would contain foundation knowledge in the biological and behavioural sciences, interpersonal and communication skills, fundamental nursing theory and practice and experience in a wide range of settings, both in hospitals and in non-institutional settings. Following successful completion of the foundation programme, students would then be able to proceed to a 'branch programme' in one of four areas: care of the adult, care of the child, care of the mentally handicapped and mental health nursing. The

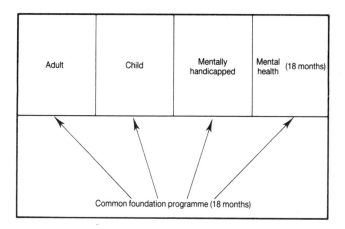

Figure 11.1 Project 2000 proposals for education leading to registration

proposal was that the branch programme would last 1 year. These times were later altered as a result of professional pressure, so that the final proposal is for a common foundation programme of 18 months followed by a further 18-month branch programme (Figure 11.1).

The standard, kind and learning outcomes of the common foundation programme have been decided by the UKCC in consultation with the four National Boards and following discussion with the profession. It is expected that rules will be issued in late 1989 to cover these points, as will guidelines to assist in the development of the curriculum, although that will remain the responsibility of the educational institution and will require approval by the appropriate National Board. National Boards have now issued guidelines for use by schools and colleges planning the new curriculum.

It is anticipated that only registration for the 'adult' branch of training will meet the current requirements of the EC Nursing Directives.

A further letter to the Statutory Bodies was issued by the Government on 10 May 1989 to deal with some of the matters not clarified in the letter of 20 May 1988 (Government letters to Miss Audrey Emerton, Chairman of the UKCC). These are as follows.

Student Service Contribution

In order to assist in manpower planning the Government suggested that students of the future should contribute not more than 1000 hours of rostered service during the 3-year programme, and that this should normally be in the third year.

All-graduate Teaching Force

Although the Government realised that an increasing proportion of the profession and its teaching staff hold degrees, they did not consider that other non-graduate teaching staff should be excluded.

Midwifery Education and Training

The Goverment expressed a welcome for the expansion of direct midwifery education and training and accepted that this should be along broadly the same lines as that for nurses in terms of supernumerary status and rostered service contribution. Shared learning with nursing students was seen as desirable, both to facilitate subsequent collaborative professional working and to maximise the use of scarce educational resources.

Entry to Nursing

The Government, while recognising steps taken to widen the entry-gate to nursing, wished to see greater practical evidence of the profession accepting vocational qualifications as satisfying the UKCC's entry requirements for nursing, this being particularly relevant for the support worker.

In addition, the Government expressed the hope that access courses to nursing would be developed in line with those established for access to higher education.

Finally, while not directly the responsibility of the Statutory bodies, efforts should be made to reduce the rigidity demonstrated by some schools and colleges of nursing regarding admission criteria.

Support Worker

This grade has the potential for attracting both young and mature entrants to the caring role, and progress to an appropriate National Council for Vocational Qualifications (NCVQ) level vocational qualification should permit access to nurse training programmes. This would also be in accordance with the Government's views on 'links and ladders' between various vocational qualifications.

The Government expressed dissatisfaction with the title 'support worker' for those working within the health-care setting and wondered if 'health-care assistant' would be more suitable. The views of the UKCC were sought on this matter.

Clarification about the respective roles of the qualified nurse and the support worker was sought.

Enrolled Nurse Training

The Government felt that, providing the steps regarding access and the support worker were taken, enrolled nurse training could cease within the next 5 years. However, where Project 2000 was implemented locally, EN training should be discontinued as part of the implementation process.

Greater flexibility in enrolled nurse conversion courses was sought by the Government, and their continued contribution to care acknowledged.

NHS REVIEW WHITE PAPER

The publication of the NHS Review White Paper (1989) had raised many anxieties regarding the continued implementation of Project 2000, and in his letter the Health Minister, Kenneth Clarke, gave three assurances:

1. 'Whatever arrangements are put in place the position of nursing, health visiting and midwifery education will be safeguarded.'
2. 'Regard will be taken of the need to maintain the momentum in implementing Project 2000.'
3. 'The Statutory Bodies will be fully involved in the work.'

At the time of writing, this letter has not received any comment. Many of the issues are not new and are part of the continuing debate. Perhaps the most contentious are those relating to the support worker grade. If the Statutory Bodies become involved in validating courses for the support worker, there is a real danger that this grade could become a 'second level' nurse under another name. On the other hand, if the Statutory Bodies do not become involved in validation of their training, this function will be undertaken by non-nurses who may not fully understand either the needs of the patients or of nursing.

Change in the Status of the Learner

Fundamental to these proposals was the requirement for the learner to be a student rather than a worker. This resulted in a recommendation that the student be supernumerary to manpower requirements for all but 6 months of the 3 years needed to obtain registration, with payment of the student by non means-tested bursaries from the Department of Health.

In June 1989 the levels of bursary were announced for the nurses starting the 13 English demonstration Project 2000 courses in the autumn of 1989. These are:

Under 26 at the start of course –	London:	£4700
	elsewhere:	£4000
Age 26 and over at the start of course –	London:	£5200
	elsewhere:	£4500

In addition to the basic/personal level of bursary there will be additions for dependents, which will be means tested on the basis of the Department of Education and Science mandatory grant rules.

Project 2000 students in receipt of bursaries were recommended not to be liable for income tax, national insurance or superannuation contributions, but like all other students would pay 20% of the personal community charge. There would be 7 weeks holiday per year.

Existing NHS staff who enter Project 2000 training, provided that they have been employed for at least 1 year, will retain their current salary rather than receive a bursary.

It was suggested that pre-registration students not on Project 2000 courses would continue to receive salaries.

It was initially hoped that midwifery would take its place as a branch programme. However, this met with opposition from a large number of midwives who felt that as midwifery was a separate profession concerned with well rather than sick women, a foundation in nursing was inappropriate. As a result, although this door was not completely closed as experimentation is possible, it was agreed that, providing it met EC requirements, midwifery should continue as an 18-month post-registration qualification and that more emphasis should be placed on securing direct entry to midwifery via a 3-year programme.

Changes in the Preparation of Nurse Teachers

It was recommended that a move should be made to achieving graduate status for all nurse teachers.

Changes in the Site of Nurse Education

In order to achieve educational currency for nursing qualifications it was recommended that schools of nursing should forge links with higher education and, where appropriate, courses should be jointly validated, for example by a National Board and either a university or the CNAA.

Manpower

In view of the 'demographic time-bomb' it was recommended that recruitment should be increased by attracting more mature students and more men. In addition it was considered that steps should be taken to widen the entry-gate to nursing education by taking account of qualifications other than the conventional Certificates of Education.

It was hoped that the changes in the educational pattern and programme would reduce wastage; this hope was based on the low wastage figures achieved by those courses offering a degree in nursing.

Despite these aims it was recognised that the qualified nurse would not be able to provide sufficient care and that there would need to be a 'helper' grade of worker. It was proposed that this person would be trained at local level to function in a specific setting.

Since these recommendations of Project 2000, other initiatives have been developed by the UK Government, which include the recognition that there are carers in a variety of settings other than health care; this has resulted in the establishment of the Support Worker, now Care, Consortium. In addition, a body has been set up to look at vocational training and to establish standards and levels of training. This body, known as the National Council for Vocational Qualifications (NCVQ), has laid down criteria for training at different levels and in advocating the development of a series of ladders by which individuals can progress to a higher level. These initiatives all have implications for the training of the health-care support worker. As already mentioned, in order to assist health authorities with the estimation of their manpower needs Price Waterhouse developed a computer manpower model. This model has been further refined by work done by Government departments attempting to produce criteria by which the 'skill mix' of staff may be determined, so that not only the number of the different grades of nurse but also the number of 'carers' may be determined.

CRITICISM OF PROJECT 2000

Despite the widespread acceptance of the proposals by the profession during the consultation stage there have been criticisms levelled at them since their final publication. Some of these focus on the assertion that the proposals are essentially an attempt to advance the professionalisation of nursing by creating an 'elite' level of nurse while much of the real work of 'caring' will be carried out by the lesser trained 'carer'. This is not in accordance with the proposals, as within the document emphasis is placed on the need for the new 'Project 2000' nurse to be a 'knowledgable doer'.

Many of the nurses presently practising realise that the training they received may not be adequate to enable them to work and compete with the nurses educated under the new system and they therefore feel threatened. This is understandable and highlights the need for concurrent updating of all grades of registered nurse. This response to change is not unexpected and is similar to the reaction to the introduction of graduates in nursing.

Nurse teachers have expressed fears regarding the links with higher education, feeling that they may be 'taken over' and disadvantaged in the broader educational setting.

The medical profession has expressed fears regarding the proposals, some of which reflect their anxiety that the nurse with a more effective level of education will not be as subservient as in the past and, therefore, less prepared to do their bidding.

Managers are concerned that the manpower predictions may not be correct and that the level of recruitment and the reduction in wastage needed to maintain the service will not be achieved. In particular, there is the fear of discontinuation in the enrolled nurse entry.

None of the criticisms and reactions are unexpected and reflect the fear that most people experience when fundamental changes are proposed, particularly when the professions involved, either directly or indirectly, are by nature traditional and conservative in outlook.

IMPLICATIONS FOR PATTERNS OF NURSE EDUCATION

The recommendations of Project 2000 necessitate a fresh approach to the pattern of nurse education. The fact that the learners will have to have experience in a wide range of clinical areas during the common foundation programme will result in fragmentation of the cohort of learners entering at any one time. This will occur because it is unlikely that any one area will be able to offer experience to a large class, so splitting into smaller groups will be needed. These small groups will progress through the required clinical experiences in one direction while others will be covering the same ground in a different order. As a result there will be great difficulty in arranging teaching timetables that allow for integration of theory with practice.

This is where some of the techniques mentioned in Part II of this book will come into their own. Remembering that the learners will be supernumerary for all of the foundation period, self-directed learning with all its variations will be the most appropriate way to progress through the theory required to provide the foundation for practice and to add explanation to experience. It may be that the large class will only rarely be together for any part of the 18 months. This may produce other problems. There is evidence to show that the support of peers plays a major part in the success of an educational programme, as shown by the way in which nurses talk of their 'set' and other groups of students of their 'class'. Maybe the smaller groups will provide this support and if this is to be allowed to develop, it is important that groups are allowed to remain intact throughout the educational period.

The links with higher education should result in some of the teachers not being nurses and, indeed, some of the teaching may take place in multidisciplinary groups. This should broaden the educational experience in a beneficial way but may also hinder the process by which the neophyte is socialised into the professional group. This is another area of challenge, which may be met by skilful mentoring and by the nurse teachers presenting as role models. This will naturally require the teachers to be able to demonstrate their clinical expertise as well as their academic knowledge. A rethink of the way in which teaching occurs in the clinical area may be needed and consideration given to ideas such as the lecturer/practitioner role and/or the establishment of some academic teaching wards and community practices. The medical profession may have much to teach nursing in this respect.

Similar challenges will arise during the branch programmes where numbers may be small in any one discipline and which will, therefore, lead to centralisation of theoretical teaching, with practice areas being spread over a number of health authorities. The variations that are likely to occur in patterns of practice will allow for interesting discussion and, it is hoped, a greater understanding of what the principles of care and the expressions of preference are. Once again, the student will need to be able to participate in the direction of learning, both in and outside the classroom.

As the outcome of these courses will produce a different type of registered nurse it is obvious that post-registration education will also have to change. This is already happening in many cases and, in particular, moves are underway to allow credit accumulation and transfer to take place, thus reducing the amount of duplication and overlap that has occurred in the past.

REFERENCES

Government Letters to Miss (later Dame) Audrey Emerton, Chairman of the UKCC, 20 May 1988 and 10 May 1989.
Government Press Release (1989) *Kenneth Clarke Announces Bursaries for Project 2000 Student Nurses*. 16 June 1989.
UKCC (1986) *Project 2000: A New Preparation for Practice*. London: UKCC.
White Paper, Review of the NHS (1989) *Working for Patients*. London: HMSO.

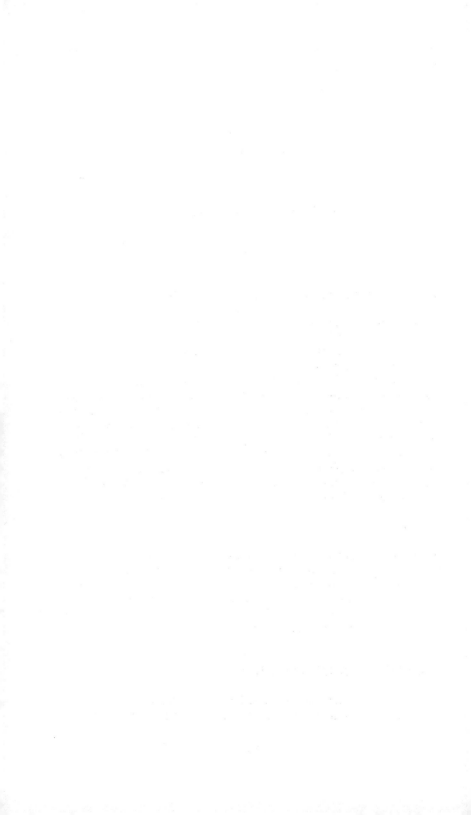

CHAPTER 12

Higher Education

POST-REGISTRATION EDUCATION

National Board Courses

Following entry to the register it is possible for students to continue their nursing education in a number of ways. The most common of these is on one of the courses in clinical nursing. These courses are in a range of areas such as care of the elderly, intensive care nursing and care of the dying patient. It will be remembered from Part I that such courses were originally under the control of the Joint Board of Clinical Nursing Studies, but since the 1979 Act they have been validated by the appropriate National Board and satisfactory completion of the course may be recorded on the UKCC Register or, if it is only a very short course, students may be given a certificate of completion.

Diploma in Nursing

This is a part-time course now conducted over 2 years. It contains studies in the biological and social sciences, theory of nursing and a nursing research project, all of greater depth than first-level programmes. These courses are held in a variety of further and/or higher education institutions but are validated by either a University or the Council for Academic Awards.

GRADUATES IN NURSING

As long ago as 1900 Mrs Bedford Fenwick stated, 'Lastly, will not Colleges of Nursing be connected with universities which will give a degree in nursing to those who satisfactorily pass through the prescribed curriculum, and so place the coping stone on the fair edifice of nursing education' (Hector, 1973). There is little doubt that she would have been astonished if she could have realised just how long it would take to establish such courses.

The first course for basic nurse preparation in a university was established in 1956 in Edinburgh as the result of efforts made by the nurse Gladys Carter, herself a graduate of an American University. She obtained money from the Rockefeller Foundation to set up a Nursing Studies Unit in the faculty of medicine, in which students taking a BSc could major in nursing and at the end of the 4½-year course obtain Registration as a general nurse. In 1959 a Diploma in Community Nursing was established at the University of Manchester and this became a Bachelor of Nursing Degree in 1969. In 1969 the University of Wales approved a 4-year course leading to a Bachelor of Nursing Degree, although the first students did not commence the course until 1972. From that point on other courses were developed in both universities and polytechnics. Not all were called nursing degrees and they were situated in varying faculties, mainly of social science or medicine. Some were 4-year courses in which nursing was integrated with the study of related disciplines such as the biological and/or social sciences; others were really a degree in an associated discipline such as sociology or psychology, with nursing theory and practice being obtained in the vacations or as a 'sandwich' within the course. All, however, enabled the graduate to obtain Registration as a nurse, either as the result of taking the State Registration examination as well as the degree examinations or as a result of the degree examinations providing exemption from the State Examination in nursing.

These courses did not meet with universal acceptance by the profession. Indeed, there was, and to some extent still is, a view held that nursing is primarily a practical skill that requires manual dexterity, a kind heart and the minimum of knowledge. This view reflects the ambivalent attitude towards graduates in nursing. At one level they are welcomed as evidence of the professionalisation of nursing and at another graduates were, and in many ways still are, feared and resented. It is a peculiar thing that while a clever doctor or lawyer is viewed with respect, the clever nurse is viewed with suspicion and expected to be 'no good practically'. Indeed, there are a number of myths associated with graduates in nursing, which, despite evidence to the contrary, still persist. These are –

in addition to 'no good practically' – 'only doing the course to enter administration', 'a failed doctor', 'not interested in patient care' and so on.

Research has been carried out that disproves all of these points. Although the new graduate may seem a little slower in practical skills than the conventionally trained nurse when first entering professional practice, there is evidence that this difference has disappeared after approximately 6 months work as a staff nurse. Ten-year follow-up studies conducted by a number of universities and polytechnics have shown not only that wastage from the profession after 10 years is low compared to nurses trained in schools of nursing (approximately 25% at 10 years for the former compared to 60% after 3 years for the latter) but also that the great majority are still employed in areas where they have direct patient/client contact. Some have entered nursing education but very few indeed have become administrators. Despite these findings the myths continue (Bircumshaw and Chapman, 1988).

Despite these myths and prejudices there is a desire among senior members of the profession for an increase in the number of graduates in nursing. This was clearly demonstrated in 1988 when the University Grants Committee's Sub-Committee, the Panel of Subjects Allied to Medicine, considered whether or not efforts should be made to acquire funding for an increase in undergraduate nurse student numbers. The four Health Departments responded positively to an enquiry as to whether or not such an increase was desirable, with the result that in 1989 it was agreed to increase undergraduate nursing numbers by 100% by the year 2000, with a 50% increase in the year 1990. This increase should result in 10% of entrants to nursing going via the university route. (These numbers do not affect the polytechnic student numbers, which are also increasing.)

What advantage is there for either the individual or the profession in having graduates in nursing? Certainly, it is not a financial advantage. There is no special pay allowance for nurses with a degree. The individual has had the benefit of a form of education that enables learning to continue throughout life, has developed problem-solving skills, has an analytical approach to situations and is able to face other health-care workers who have also undergone university preparation on an equal footing. The profession benefits from having within it individuals who are questioning in approach, less likely to carry out traditional patterns of care, able to use and/or carry out research and able to compete nationally and internationally in all health-care settings. Margaret Scott Wright, the first professor of nursing in the UK, said in her inaugural lecture, 'A viable profession is going to depend increasingly on its ability to adapt to meet changes in the social, economic and scientific environment. Thus it will require in its ranks those who are able to question accepted customs and practice, to establish scientific principles of clinical practice and manpower organisation . . . such objectives are going to depend more and more on the preparation of some nurses to undertake research into professional practice and procedures' (Scott-Wright, 1968).

The need for nurses to undertake research into nursing practice has been and still is a fundamental responsibility of university departments of nursing, although not restricted to them. Indeed, the first systematic approach to nursing research commenced in the 1960s in the Royal College of Nursing as a result of money given by the Department of Health.

Now most courses contain research appreciation and many require students to conduct small-scale research projects. Unfortunately, all this activity has not had the impact on practice that might have been expected. The reasons for this are varied and range from ignorance of the research that has been carried out to disbelief of the findings and a fundamental feeling that what has always been done is good enough for present practice.

Following the establishment of direct entry to nursing undergraduate courses many other courses have been developed in higher education to allow nurses to study for first or higher degrees and to enable research degrees to be obtained.

There are, of course, other graduates who enter nursing having obtained degrees in a wide variety of subjects. There is a facility for such graduates to take a shortened course leading to Registration, although many choose to take the 3-year course.

A more unusual route to graduation has developed from the Diploma in Nursing. Nurses who successfully complete the diploma may then be eligible to undertake a further 2-year part-time study leading to a degree.

CREDIT ACCUMULATION AND TRANSFER

This is a method by which students can obtain credit for a wide variety of courses taken in institutions, by distance learning methods and, in some cases, in clinical settings. The summation of these credits can be equated first to a certificate and then a diploma and can provide entry to a degree programme.

The different countries of the UK have, via their National Boards, developed similar approaches to continuing education. For example, Scotland has a well-established Diploma in Professional Studies, while Wales describes its programme as a Framework for the Development of Professional Practice.

The National Health Service Training Authority has developed a variety of courses, mainly in Colleges of Further Education, some of which involve shared learning between social work students and nurses undertaking courses in the care of the mentally handicapped. This collaboration between the Statutory Body for Social Work (the Council for the Education and Training of Social Workers) and nursing's Statutory Bodies (National Boards) is a welcome development.

Other links with higher education are likely to develop as a result of the implementation of the proposals of Project 2000, all of which should serve to place nursing education firmly in the mainstream of education and ensure that qualifications gained within the profession have a wider educational currency than in the past.

The overall effect of these changes is that, in future, a greatly increased number of nurses will be graduates, either of nursing or other disciplines. Such people are more likely to demand a say in their education, both in content and process, and when working within the profession may be less tolerant of the status quo. This increase in the number of people with educated minds and a greater understanding of research findings should result in improved standards of care and also an increase in professionalism.

REFERENCES

Bircumshaw D and Chapman C M (1988a) A follow-up of the graduates of the Cardiff Bachelor of Nursing Degree Course. *Journal of Advanced Nursing*, **13**: 273–279.

Bircumshaw D and Chapman C M (1988b) A study to compare the practice style of graduate and non-graduate nurses and midwives: the pilot study. *Journal of Advanced Nursing*, **13**: 605–614.

Hector W (1973) *Mrs Bedford-Fenwick*. London: RCN.

Scott-Wright M (1968) Inaugural lecture, Department of Nursing Studies, Edinburgh University.

Bibliography

Abercrombie M L J (1974) *Aims and Techniques of Group Teaching*. London: Society for Research into Higher Education.

Abrami P, Leenthal L and Perry R (1982) Educational seduction. *Review of Educational Research*, **52**: 446–464.

Allan D M E, Grosswald S J and Means R P (1984) Facilitating self-directed learning. In: *Continuing Education for the Health Professions: Developing, Managing and Evaluating Programs for Maximum Impact on Patient Care*, Green J S, Grosswald S J, Suter E and Walthall D B (eds.). San Francisco, California: Jossey Bass.

Archambault R D (ed.) (1964) *John Dewey on Education: Selected Writings*. New York: Random House.

Argyris C (1982) *Reasoning, Learning and Action*. San Francisco, California: Jossey Bass.

Argyris C and Schon D (1974) *Theory in Practice: Increasing Professional Effectiveness*. San Francisco, California: Jossey Bass.

Austin E K (1981) *Guidelines for the Development of Continuing Education Offerings for Nurses*. Norwalk, Connecticut: Appleton-Century-Crofts.

Bales R F (1950) *Interaction Process Analysis: A Method for the Study of Small Groups*. Cambridge, Massachusetts: Addison-Wesley.

Beckett C (1984) Student status in nursing: a discussion on the status of the student and how it affects training. *Journal of Advanced Nursing*, **9**: 363–374.

Belbin E and Belbin R M (1972) *Problems in Adult Retraining*. London: Heinemann.

Bendall E R D (1975) *So You Passed Nurse*. London: Royal College of Nursing.

Bligh D (1971) *What's the Use of Lectures?* Harmondsworth: Penguin.

Bolton E B (1980) A conceptual analysis of the mentoring relationship in the career development of women. *Adult Education*, **30**: 195–207.

Boot R and Reynolds M (1983) *Learning and Experience in Formal Education*. Manchester Monograph. Manchester: Department of Adult and Higher Education, University of Manchester.

Botkin J, Elmandjra M and Malitza M (1979) *No Limits to Learning: Bridging the Human Gap.* London: Pergamon.

Boud D (ed.) (1973) *Experiential Learning Techniques in Higher Education.* Human Potential Learning Project. Guildford, Surrey: University of Surrey.

Boud D J (ed.) (1981) *Developing Student Autonomy in Learning.* London: Kogan Page.

Boud D and Prosser M T (1980) Sharing responsibility: staff–student cooperation in learning. *British Journal of Educational Technology*, 11(1): 24–35.

Boud D, Keogh R and Walker M (1985) *Reflection: Turning Experience into Learning.* London: Kogan Page.

Bower G H and Hilgard E R (1981) *Theories of Learning*, 5th edn. Englewood Cliffs, New Jersey: Prentice Hall.

Bridges W (1973) The three faces of humanistic education. In: *Curriculum Development*, Orlosky D E and Smith B O. Rand McNally, Chicago: Issues and Insights.

Brocket R and Hiemstra R (1985) Bridging the theory–practice gap in self-directed learning. In *Self-Directed Learning: From Theory to Practice*, Brookfield S D (ed.). New Directions for Continuing Education No. 25. San Francisco, California: Jossey Bass.

Brown A (1979) *Groupwork.* London: Heinemann.

Brown B J (1984) The Dean as mentor. *Nursing Health Care*, 5(2): 88–91.

Brown G (1971) *Human Teaching for Human Learning.* New York: Viking Press.

Brown I B (ed.) (1975) *The Live Classroom.* California: Esalen/Viking.

Brundage D H and Mackeracher D (1980) *Adult Learning Principles and their Application to Program Planning.* Ontario: Ministry of Education.

Bruner J S (1966) *Towards a Theory of Instruction.* Cambridge, Massachusetts: Bleknap.

Burnard P (1985) The teacher as facilitator. *Senior Nurse*, 3(1): 34–37.

Carpenter M (1978) Managerialism and the division of labour in nursing. In: *Readings in the Sociology of Nursing*, Dingwall R and McIntosh J (eds.). Edinburgh: Churchill Livingstone.

Chene A (1983) The concept of autonomy in adult education: a philosophical discussion. *Adult Education Quarterly*, 32(1): 38–47.

Clark M (1978) Meeting the needs of the adult learner: using non-formal education for social action. *Convergence*, XI: 3–4.

Clawson J G (1985) Is mentoring necessary? *Training and Development Journal*, 39(4): 36–39.

Clift J C and Imrie B W (1981) *Assessing Students and Appraising Teaching.* London: Croom Helm.

Clutterbuck D (1985) *Everybody Needs a Mentor: How To Further Talent within an Organisation.* London: The Institute of Personnel Management.

Coleman J S (1982) Experiential learning and information assimilation: towards an appropriate mix. *Child and Youth Services*, 14(3–4): 12–20.

Collins N W (1983) *Professional Women and Their Mentors.* Englewood Cliffs, New Jersey: Prentice Hall.

Conrad D and Hedin D (1982) The impact of experiential education on adolescent development. *Child and Youth Services*, **4**(3–4): 57–76.

Cross K P (1981) *Adults as Learners*. San Francisco, California: Jossey Bass.

Cross-Durrant A (1984) Lifelong education in the writings of John Dewey. *International Journal of Lifelong Education*, **3**(2): 115–125.

Cunningham P M (1983) Helping students extract meaning from experience. In: *Helping Adults Learn how To Learn*, Smith R M (ed.). New Directions for Continuing Education No. 19. San Francisco, California: Jossey Bass.

Darkenwald G G and Merriam S B (1982) *Adult Education: Foundations of Practice*. New York: Harper and Row.

Darling L W (1986) What to do about toxic mentors. *Nurse Educator*, **11**(2): 29–30.

Davis B (ed.) (1987) *Nursing Education: Research and Developments*. London: Croom Helm.

Davis C M (1981) Affective education for the health professions. *Physical Therapy*, **61**(11): 1587–1593.

Douglas T (1976) *Groupwork Practice*. London: Tavistock.

Dowd C (1983) Learning through experience. *Nursing Times*, 27 July: 50–52.

Du Bois E E (1982) Human resource development: expanding role. In: *Materials and Methods in Adult and Continuing Education*, Klevens C (ed.). Canoga Park, California: Klevins Publications.

Edmunds M (1983) The nurse preceptor role. *Nurse Practitioner*, **8**(6): 52–53.

Elias J L (1979) Andragogy revisited. *Adult Education*, **29**: 252–256.

Elias J L and Merriam S (1980) *Philosophical Foundations of Adult Education*. Florida: Krieger.

English National Board for Nursing, Midwifery and Health Visiting (1985) *ENB Approval Process for Courses in Nursing, Midwifery and Health Visiting*. London: ENB.

Erikson-Megel M (1985) New faculty in nursing: socialisation and the role of the mentor. *Journal of Nursing Education*, **24**(7): 303–305.

Fagan M M and Fagan P D (1983) Mentoring among nurses. *Nursing Health Care*, **4**(2): 77–82.

Fagan M M and Walter G (1982) Mentoring among teachers. *Journal of Educational Research*, **76**(2): 113–118.

Famighetti R A (1981) Experiential learning: the close encounters of the institutional kind. *Gerontology and Geriatric Education*, **2**(2): 129–132.

Fox F E (1983) The spiritual core of experiential education. *Journal of Experiential Education*, **16**(1): 3–6.

Freire P (1985) *The Politics of Education*. South Hadley, Massachusetts: Bergin and Garvey.

Fretwell J E (1982) *Ward Teaching and Learning*. London: RCN.

Gager R (1982) Experiential education: strengthening the learning process. *Child and Youth Services*, **4**(3–4): 31–39.

Gallego A P (1983) *Evaluating the School*. London: RCN.

George P and Kummerow J (1981) Mentoring for career women. *Training*, **18**(2): 44–49.

Guba E G (1978) *Towards a Methodology of Naturalistic Inquiry in Educational Evaluation*. SE Monograph Series in Evaluation No. 8. University of California, Los Angeles: Center for the Study of Evaluation.

Hamilton M S (1981) Mentorhood: a key to nursing leadership. *Nursing Leadership*, **4**(1): 4–13.

Hamrick M and Stone C (1979) Promoting experiential learning. *Health Education*, **10**(4): 38–41.

Hare A P (1976) *Handbook of Small Group Research*. New York: Free Press.

Hendricks G and Fadiman J (eds.) (1976) *Transpersonal Education: A Curriculum for Feeling and Being*. Englewood Cliffs, New Jersey: Prentice Hall.

Heron J (1973) *Experience and Method*. Human Potential Research Project. Guildford, Surrey: University of Surrey.

Heron J (1981) *Experiential Research: A New Paradigm*. Human Potential Research Project. Guildford, Surrey: University of Surrey.

Hinchliff S M (ed.) (1979) *Teaching in Clinical Nursing*. Edinburgh: Churchill Livingstone.

Holt R (1982) An alternative to mentorship. *Adult Education*, **55**(2): 152–156.

Houle C O (1972) *The Design of Learning*. San Francisco, California: Jossey Bass.

Houle C O (1984) *Patterns of Learning*. San Francisco, California: Jossey Bass.

Hudson A (1983) The politics of experiential learning. In: *Learning and Experience in Formal Education*, Boot R and Reynolds M. Manchester Monograph. Manchester: Department of Adult and Higher Education, University of Manchester.

Hunter E (1972) *Encounter in the Classroom*. New York: Holt Reinhart and Winston.

Jarvis P (1983) *The Theory and Practice of Adult and Continuing Education*. London: Croom Helm.

Jarvis P (1985) *The Sociology of Adult and Continuing Education*. London: Croom Helm.

Jarvis P (1987) *Adult Learning in the Social Context*. London: Croom Helm.

Jenkins D and Shipman M D (1976) *Curriculum: An Introduction*. London: Open Books.

Kanter R M (1979) *Men and Women of the Corporation*. New York: Basic Books.

Kidd J R (ed.) (1973) *How Adults Learn*. Chicago: Association Press.

Klopf G J and Harrison J (1981) Moving up the career ladder: the case for mentors. *Principal*, **61**(1): 41–43.

Knox A B (1977) *Adult Development and Learning: A Handbook on Individual Growth and Competence in the Adult Years*. San Francisco, California: Jossey Bass.

Knox A B (ed.) (1980) *Teaching Adults Effectively*. San Francisco, California: Jossey Bass.

Legge D (1982) *The Education of Adults in Britain*. Milton Keynes: Open University Press.

Levison R H (1979) Experiential education abroad. *Teaching Sociology*, **6**(4): 415–419.

Lewin K (1969) Quasi-stationary social equilibria and the problems of permanent change. In: *The Planning of Change*, Bennis W G, Benn K D and Chin R (eds.). New York: Holt Reinhart and Winston.

Lipsett L and Avakian N A (1981) Assessing experiential learning: lifelong learning. *The Adult Years*, **5**(2): 18–22.

Lomas P (1973) *True and False Experience*. London: Allen Lane.

McCamiele R (ed.) (1982) *Calling Education into Account*. London: Heinemann.

McCormick R and James M (1983) *Curriculum Evaluation in Schools*. London: Croom Helm.

McIntosh A (1982) Psychology and adult education. In: *Psychology in Practice*, Canter S and Canter D (eds.). Chichester: John Wiley and Sons.

Marshall E K and Kurtz P D (eds.) (1982) *Interpersonal Helping Skills: A Guide to Training Methods, Programs and Resources*. San Francisco, California: Jossey Bass.

Martin J R (1970) *Explaining, Understanding and Teaching*. New York: McGraw Hill.

Menson B (ed.) (1982) *Building on Experiences in Adult Development*. New Directions for Experiential Learning No. 16. San Francisco, California: Jossey Bass.

Merriam S (1984) Mentors and proteges: a critical review of the literature. *Adult Education Quarterly*, **33**(3): 161–173.

Mezeiro J (1981) A critical theory of adult learning and education. *Adult Education*, **32**(1): 3–24.

Mouton J S and Blake R R (1984) *Synergogy: A New Strategy for Education, Training and Development*. San Francisco, California: Jossey Bass.

Nadler L (ed.) (1984) *The Handbook of Human Resource Development*. New York: John Wiley and Sons.

Niebuhr H (1977) *Revitalizing American Education: A New Approach that Might Just Work*. Belmont, California: Wadsworth.

Noble P (1983) *Formation of Freirian Facilitators*. Chicago: Latino Institute.

Nuttall P (1982) Take me to your mentor. *Nursing Times*, **78**(20): 826.

Nyberg D (ed.) (1975) *The Philosophy of Open Education*. London: Routledge and Kegan Paul.

Osborn T (1984) The question of peer assessment: self and society. *European Journal of Humanistic Psychology*, **XII**(4): 201–206.

Patton M Q (1982) *Practical Evaluation*. Beverly Hills, California: Sage.

Phillip-Jones L (1982) *Mentors and Proteges*. New York: Arbour House.

Rawlings M E and Rawlings L (1983) Mentoring and networking for helping professionals. *Personnel and Guidance Journal*, **62**(2): 116–118.

Ringuette E L (1983) A note on experiential learning in professional training. *Journal of Clinical Psychology*, **39**(2): 302–304.

Roche G R (1979) Much ado about mentors. *Harvard Business Review*, **56**: 14–28.

Rogers C R (1972) The facilitation of significant learning. In: *The Psychology of Open Learning and Teaching: An Inquiry Approach*, Silberman L, Allender J S and Yanoff J M. Boston, Massachussets: Little Brown and Co.

Rogers J (ed.) (1977) *Adults Learning*. Milton Keynes: Open University Press.

Rogers J C (1982) Sponsorship – developing leaders for occupational therapy. *American Journal of Occupational Therapy*, **36**: 309–313.

Rogers J and Groombridge B (1976) *Right to Learn: The Case for Adult Equality*. London: Arrow.

Schafer B P and Morgan M K (1980) An experiential learning laboratory: a new dimension in teaching mental health skills. *Issues in Mental Health Nursing*, **2**(3): 47–57.

Schmidt J A and Wolfe J S (1980) The mentor partnership: discovery of professionalism. *NASPA Journal*, **17**: 45–51.

Schon D A (1983) *The Reflective Practitioner: How Professionals Think in Action*. New York: Basic Books.

Schorr T M (1978) The lost art of mentoring. *American Journal of Nursing*, **78**: 1873.

Shamian J and Inhaber R (1985) The concept and practice of preceptorship in contemporary nursing: a review of pertinent literature. *The International Journal of Nursing Studies*, **22**(2): 79–88.

Shapiro E C, Haseltime F and Rowe M (1978) Moving up: role models, mentors and the patron system. *Sloan Management Review*, **19**: 51–58.

Shropshire C O (1981) Group experiential learning in adult education. *The Journal of Continuing Education in Nursing*, **12**(6): 5–9.

Simon S B, Howe L W and Kirschenbaum H (1978) *Values Clarification*, revised edn. New York: A and W Visual Library.

Sockett H (1976) *Designing the Curriculum*. London: Open Books.

Soth N (1981) Experiential education from a cultural viewpoint: the peer evaluation meeting as a ritual of enculturation. *Alternative Higher Education*, **6**(2): 88–95.

Speizer J J (1981) Role models, mentors and sponsors: the elusive concept. *Signs*, **6**: 692–712.

Stenhouse L (1975) *An Introduction to Curriculum Research and Development*. London: Heinemann.

Stitch T F (1983) Experiential therapy. *Journal of Experiential Education*, **5**(3): 23–30.

Taylor S (1986) Mentors: who are they and what are they doing? *Thrust for Educational Leadership*, **15**(7): 39–41.

Tough A M (1982) *Intentional Changes; A Fresh Approach to Helping People Change*. New York: Cambridge Books.

Wlodkowski R J (1985) *Enhancing Adult Motivation to Learn*. San Francisco, California: Jossey Bass.

Index